Contents

Acknowledgements

The author wishes to express his gratitude to all those who have provided the inspiration, advice and practical assistance in the writing of this book. In particular he would like to thank:

June Young, for her advice and assistance in preparing the drafts of the manuscript; my wife Barbara and my family for their encouragement, and my granddaughter, Matilda; Dr Tom Smith, for his example and encouragement; Vivenne Freeman for her unfailing support; Debbie Kelley, for her assistance in preparing the illustrations and diagrams; Dane Woodruff and the staff of Health Trust Alliance ®; Garth and Mary Young for their lifelong friendship, support and encouragement; Samuel Hahnemann, whose birthday the author shares and whose life and work have inspired him; faculty members, tutors, students and staff of the British Institute of Homo-eopathy world-wide with whom the author is proud to be associated; William and Beth Tankard-Hahnemann for their selfless support and friendship; the staff of The Crowood Press Ltd and David Warkentin.

Foreword

This remarkable book covers, probably for the first time under one cover, every facet of homoeopathy, old and new, central or peripheral, accepted or contentious.

From the writings of the ancient philosophers to our current understanding of the philosophy and principles of homoeopathy, from classical to applied homoeopathy in the whole spectrum of homoeopathic treatments. From chronic miasmic conditions to those arising from modern urban pollution and environmental stress, its scope includes advice on the exposure of homeopathic remedies to harmful rays in airport security checks.

In a logical manner Dr. Cook has presented his knowledge and experience based on fifteen years in conventional medicine and twenty-five years in homoeopathic medicine in research, manufacture, teaching and practice.

I am sure that readers will be stimulated and their appreciation of homoeopathy will be refreshed, expanded and renewed. I thoroughly recommend this book to practitioners and students alike.

William Tankard-Hahnemann
Sussex, 1999

CHAPTER 1
Origins and History of Homoeopathic Medicine

From the ancient philosophers to a credible, scientific alternative therapy. Samuel Hahnemann, founder of modern homoeopathy. Its rise and development. Its decline and re-birth in the twentieth century to establish itself as an intrinsic part of the whole fabric of modern medicine worldwide.

BIRTH OF MODERN HOMOEOPATHIC MEDICINE

It was early in the year 1790. Dr Samuel Hahnemann was seated at a small, candle-lit table, set behind a curtain in the corner of the ill-heated room where his wife and family of five children were sleeping. He usually worked on his translations of medical and scientific works until 4 or 5 o'clock in the morning, but this night it was different.

He had been taking 'as an experiment' two doses of the drug Cinchona (Peruvian bark). He already knew that the drug induced some kind of fever if taken in relatively large doses. He recorded his reactions as follows:

My feet and fingertips, etc., at first became cold. I became languid and drowsy; then my heart began to palpitate; my pulse became quick and hard; I developed an intolerable anxiety and trembling with prostration in all my limbs; pulsation in the head; redness of cheeks and thirst.

Briefly, these were all the symptoms associated with intermittent fever [malaria]; all made their appear-ance. These symptoms lasted from two to three hours every time and recurred only when I repeated the dose. When I discontinued the medicine I was once more in good health.

The remarkable fact was, however, that the drug he had taken – Cinchona – was used extensively for the *treatment* of malaria.

Indeed, Cinchona had attracted Samuel Hahnemann's interest in the first place since it was one of the few drugs known at that time to be effective in the treatment of a disease. Thus he recognized that Cinchona, which was effective in the treatment of malaria, induced similar symptoms to this disease when taken by a healthy person.

In another note, he recorded:

Peruvian bark (*Cinchona officinalis*) which is used as a remedy for intermittent fever (malaria) acts because it can produce symptoms similar to those of intermittent fever in healthy people. Similia Similibus Curentur – let likes be cured by likes.

In this epoch-making experiment Samuel Hahnemann had established the basic fundamental principle of his new therapy that

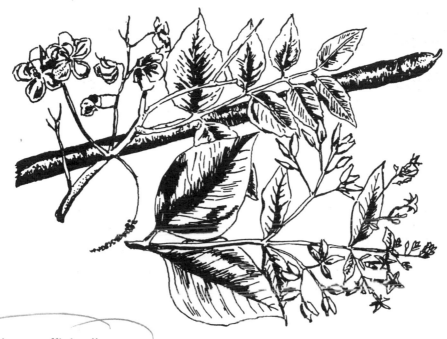

Cinchona officinalis

he named homoeopathy. A new era in medicine had begun, which was to rock the reactionary medical establishment to its foundations and give rise to a bitter conflict that exists in some quarters even today.

Samuel Hahnemann – Founder of Modern Homoeopathy

Christian Friedrich Samuel was born shortly before midnight on Thursday 10 April 1755, the second son of Christian and Johanna Hahnemann. His birthplace was Meissen, the small picturesque town on the River Elbe in eastern Germany, with its high-gabled roofs crowded along the lower slopes of the Erz mountains. Soon to be known simply as Samuel Hahnemann, he was brought up under the stern but kindly eye of his father, an artist at the famous Meissen porcelain factory during a period punctuated by the hardships of the Seven Years War which raged across Saxony from 1756 to 1763.

Samuel soon demonstrated his exceptional ability. At the age of twelve, he was teaching other pupils the rudiments of Greek and eventually spoke eleven languages fluently. It was this linguistic ability that was to influence his life and the course of medicine in later years.

He entered the University of Leipzig at Easter 1775 to study medicine, having given a masterly dissertation in Latin entitled *The Anatomy of the Human Hand* to graduate from the Prince's School in Meissen.

Maintaining a meagre subsistence by translating papers from Greek into English and German for other students, and taking the place of absent students in their 'eating house', which was rather like a soup kitchen, Hahnemann soon questioned the wisdom of the early teaching of contemporary medicine he had received.

He became so disenchanted that he attended lectures in chemistry instead – a science to which he made a significant contribution in later years. His frustration was increased by the total lack of clinical facilities. His comment in a student journal that, in his view, 'more people died of their treatment than their diseases' alienated his tutors and the head of the medical school Professor Clarus, and led inevitably to Hahnemann's withdrawal from the University at the end of his first academic year.

Medical Reform

After his acrimonious departure from the University of Leipzig, Hahnemann spent a year in Vienna at the general hospital in an attempt to gain the clinical experience denied to him. He then spent a few months working for the Governor of Transylvania (now part of Hungary) before taking up residence at the University of Erlangan in Bavaria where he gained the degree of Doctor of Medicine in August 1779.

Before even gaining his degree, Hahnemann had embarked on a campaign for medical reform which he was to continue for the rest of his long life. Indeed, had he not established his new system of medicine – the Healing Art of Homoeopathy – he would have undoubtedly been remembered for his work in reforming orthodox medicine, which he saw as stagnant, barbaric, ineffective and totally lacking in any scientific basis.

Based on purging techniques 'to draw the disease from the body', eighteenth and nineteenth-century medicine relied heavily on venesection, blood-letting or cupping. Copious withdrawals of blood were considered to be urgently necessary by generations of physicians for most diseases and even for pregnant women.

The notable French physician, Broussais, for example, believed it to be so indispensable that he called for failure to carry out venesection to be treated as a punishable offence. Other forms of purging – massive enemas, violent laxatives and stomach-wrenching emetics were also employed. If the patient, thus debilitated, survived this onslaught, massive doses of toxic nostrums were given – elixirs, bilge water, eye of the toad, oil of cajeput or asafoetida (a resinous gum) and many more were given, followed perhaps by a hot iron applied to the crotch!

For more than sixty years, Samuel Hahnemann produced a constant stream of articles and essays attacking these diabolical practices. 'Blood letting, fever remedies, tepid baths, lowering drinks, everlasting aperiants and clysters form the vicious circle in which the German physician turns', he wrote.

To the draconian physicians, Hahnemann's quest for a humanized, compassionate and gentle approach to medical treatment was anathema. Medical practice had undergone no radical change in the eighteenth century and was rooted in tradition. The teaching of medicine was characterized by rigid conformity with accepted practice with no scientific principles and was rooted in superstition and quackery. He lived, however, to see medical treatment undergo a metamorphosis when the last bastions of blood-letting fell to enlightened opinion and the homoeopathic approach was interwoven in the entire fabric of medical practice.

DEVELOPMENT OF HOMOEOPATHY

After practising in the poor copper mining town of Hettstedt in 1780–81, then in the larger town of Dessau where he met and married his first wife Johanna in 1782, and finally the rural community of Gommern, Samuel Hahnemann virtually withdrew from medicine.

His experiences had only served to convince him of the futility of orthodox medical practice and his verbal and written attacks on its shortcomings had alienated his contemporaries. Thus withdrawn, he embarked on seemingly aimless travels over the next fifteen years, staying in no less than twenty towns along the route of the River Elbe from Hamburg in the north to Dresden in the south.

No longer practising, he maintained himself and his growing family by translating medical and scientific works for two publishers, one in Leipzig and the other in Dresden, from English, French, Spanish, Greek or Latin into his native German.

His travels eventually brought him in 1790 to the village of Stotteritz on the outskirts of Leipzig where he lived in one room with his impoverished family. It was here that he carried out the experiment with Cinchona which was to end his search for a safe, gentle and compassionate alternative medical therapy system.

Dr Dudgeon (1854) wrote an account of Hahnemann's life at Stotteritz:

> After toiling all night at his task of translating works for the press, he frequently assisted his brave-hearted wife to wash the family clothes during the day and as they were unable to purchase soap they employed raw potatoes for this purpose. The quantity of bread he was able to earn by his writing for his large family was so small that he had to weigh out to each an equal portion.

He abhorred the cruel practices that prevailed, the incompetence, the hypocrisy, the quackery and the indifference to the suffering of the patient. He espoused the value of proper diet, sanitation, cleanliness, personal hygiene, exercise and fresh air.

His views were encapsulated in his book entitled *The Friend of Health*, published in Leipzig in 1795. Set against contemporary medical knowledge and living conditions, Hahnemann was years ahead of his time.

Pharmacy

Calling on his experience and knowledge of chemistry, Hahnemann penned his *Pharmaceutical Lexicon*, published in four volumes in 1793. He instructed, *inter alia*, that tinctures should be prepared from fresh, clean plant materials, that poisons should be kept under lock and key, that batches should be properly labelled and procedures carried out in a reliable manner with clear safety instructions. It is remarkable that many of his provisions are now incorporated in the Medicines Acts of England and Wales in 1968 and 1971 and similar legislation in other developed countries governing Current Good Manufacturing Practice (CGMP) today.

Having enunciated the basic principle of homoeopathy, Hahnemann developed his understanding of the true nature of disease and the natural principles of cure, bringing these principles together to introduce his new system of the Healing Art.

The Organon of Medicine

The first edition of Samuel Hahnemann's quintessential work, *The Organon of Rational Healing* (*Organon der Rationellen Heilkunde*), was published in Dresden in 1810. Later he changed the title to *The Organon of the Healing Art*. The year 1810 is now regarded by homoeopaths as the year of birth of homoeopathy as it is known today.

The Organon of Medicine, as it is now generally known, ran to six editions in

9

Hahnemann's lifetime and has been translated into eleven languages. No training in homoeopathy is complete without proper study of the *Organon* and a detailed study is presented in following chapters of this book.

Materia Medica Pura

Having established homoeopathy on a scientific basis, based on the Cinchona experiment – the 'first homoeopathic medicine' – Hahnemann needed more homoeopathic medicines to demonstrate its clinical effectiveness over a wide range of disease conditions.

He set out on a laborious programme of what he termed 'provings' (German verb, prüfen – to test) to introduce a series of homoeopathic remedies.

Following the basic homoeopathic principle, a range of natural substances – animal, vegetable and mineral – were given to healthy people (provers). The disease symptoms thus induced – the so-called proving symptoms – were by the homoeopathic 'like with like' principle, indicative that the given substance had potential use as a homoeopathic remedy.

Hahnemann carried out many provings on his own body, often driving himself to the brink of serious illness by taking large material doses of toxic substances. It is clear from his letters to his fellow provers that he regarded this work as a duty for the benefit of humankind. Subsequently, he conscripted members of his family, friends and a growing number of physicians who became his followers.

Over the ten years following the publication of the *Organon*, he proved about 200 remedies, the details of which he published in his *Materia Medica Pura* in four volumes, between 1811 and 1821. The format of this *Materia Medica* and others that followed are discussed in subsequent chapters.

The Chronic Diseases

Hahnemann's other great work was written later in his life, shortly before his first retirement. *The Chronic Diseases: Their Peculiar Nature and Their Homoeopathic Cure* was published in 1832. He discussed his philosophy and the fundamentals of medicine, seeking to find a rational explanation. In the second volume of the book he introduced seventy-nine new homoeopathic medicines. *The Chronic Diseases* was contentious, however, and led to much criticism from his contemporaries, particularly his 'psora theory' and the fact that his new remedies were presented on the basis of clinical evidence rather than provings.

Constantine Hering – architect of homoeopathy in America

Although it was Dr Hans Burch Gram, the immigrant son of a Danish sea captain, who first set up the homoeopathic practice in America – in New York in 1828 – the true architect of homoeopathy across the American nation was Dr Constantine Hering who arrived in the country five years later. He established the infrastructure from which homoeopathy grew in America to its position today.

Constantine Hering was born in Saxony in the town of Oschatz on 1 January 1800. Oschatz has since been rebuilt, but in Hering's day it resembled Hahnemann's birthplace in Meissen, which is situated only a few miles away. Constantine's father was a headmaster at the local school and also a church organist and he often played to crowded churches in Leipzig. He was also known as *Magister* – a title signifying Master of Arts. The story may be apocryphal but it was said that Constantine's father was playing his organ in the New Year when word reached him that his wife had given birth to a son. He burst forth with the strains of the much-loved German carol *Nun Danket* (*Now Thank We All Our God*).

Like Samuel Hahnemann he grew up in a well-disciplined family and he showed great respect and affection for his parents. In his home there were high moral standards, industry, sobriety, orderliness and piety. Constantine decided very early in life to study medicine and at the age of eighteen he commenced studying medicine at the University of Leipzig as Hahnemann himself had done. His ambition was nearly thwarted when, dissecting the exhumed body of a suicide, he sustained a wound to the forefinger of his right hand and the finger became infected. Conventional contemporary treatments were given including, inevitably, venesection through blood leeches, calomel and silver nitrate. Amputation was finally advised.

On the advice of a local homoeopathic physician who had been a student of Samuel Hahnemann he took the homoeopathic remedy Arsenicum album, although he had little faith in its ability to cure, particularly, as he put it at the time, it was in a 'ridiculously small dose'. After a few doses, however, he found a complete cure Many years later he wrote of Samuel Hahnemann who had 'saved my finger ... I have devoted my whole hand to the promulgation of his teaching – not only my hand but my entire mind, body and soul'.

Unfortunately the head of the medical school in Leipzig at that time was the same arch enemy of Samuel Hahnemann, Professor Clarus, and whilst studying in his final year for his doctorate of medicine, Professor Clarus instructed him to write an essay on the ineffectiveness of homoeopathy and to refute its principles.

Hering commenced the project but on studying the principles of homoeopathy he came to accept that homoeopathy was a true art of healing. In his dilemma he wrote to Samuel Hahnemann to ask for his advice and to offer his services as a prover of homoeopathic medicines.

Being a pragmatist Samuel Hahnemann replied to Constantine Hering:

> As you wish to gain a doctor's degree in medicine next Spring I beg and counsel you not to allow your homoeopathic opinions to be known by the allopathic physicians of Leipzig, least of all by Professor Clarus, if you do not wish to be rejected at your examination. Yet when you have your degree then fear nothing from the obstacles that will be put in your way. I have confidence in you.

Constantine Hering, being a man of high principles, did not take Hahnemann's advice and did not complete his thesis, thus ruining his chances of gaining his degree at Leipzig. He subsequently left Leipzig for the University of Wuetzburg where he obtained his doctorate of medicine on 22 March 1826. Again, like Hahnemann, Constantine Hering suffered from poverty during his stay in Wuetzburg, eating in a free eating house. The hard, stale rye bread he was given, he would soak in weak broth as the crusts were so hard they caused his gums to bleed. Many years later Hering told how he had been ridiculed by his fellow students because of his belief in homoeopathy.

Some months later he left for a tour of South America where he was planning to conduct medical research. Although he had not met Hahnemann personally Hering became a close friend and a loyal follower through their correspondence during the last fifteen years of Hahnemann's life.

Constantine Hering spent five years in South America and during this time proved several new homoeopathic remedies, including *Spigelia*, *Theridion* and, importantly, *Lachesis*. These remedies have proved to be of great value in the alleviation of suffering.

He also proved the remedy, *Hepar Sulphuris*. Hahnemann had already proved this remedy but Hering was able to verify his findings and expand on the proving symptoms. It was said that while proving Lachesis, which is prepared from the venom of the very poisonous Bushmaster (Suruku) snake, Hering enlisted the help of his wife to write down the details of his reactions to the drug.

She also had the antidote and as he became progressively weaker and close to death she begged him to let her give him the antidote. In the process of proving this drug by taking ever increasing quantities his left arm became paralysed and remained so for the rest of his life.

In 1833 Dr Constantine Hering emigrated to the United States of America. It was Hering who created the whole infrastructure of homoeopathy that enabled it to grow in America, whilst Dr Gram simply practised homoeopathy, which, although worthy, did little to spread homoeopathy throughout the country.

Dr Hering finally settled in Pennsylvania and along with Dr Detweiler (who in 1828 had become the first physician to practise there), Dr Hering established the North American Academy of Homoeopathic Healing Art in Allentown in Pennsylvania – the first centre of homoeopathic learning in America.

In March 1841 Samuel Hahnemann wrote to Constantine Hering in Philadelphia requesting that he grant his second wife, Melanie, a Diploma in Homoeopathy from the Allentown Academy as she held no formal qualification. In spite of their friendship, Hering refused Hahnemann's request.

Until his death Hahnemann corresponded regularly with Dr Hering in Philadelphia. Constantine Hering, was the first person to suggest the use of nosodes (see Chapter 7) in homoeopathy and in 1833 he introduced Lyssin from the saliva of a mad dog as a homoeopathic remedy. His work in this area influenced others in Europe, including Dr Weber, who prepared *Anthrocinum* from the spleen of animals affected by anthrax.

Constantine Hering founded the American Institute of Homoeopathy (AIH) in 1835 and was elected its first President. The AIH is the oldest medical professional body in America!

In 1836, he established a second college – the Homoeopathic Medical College of Pennsylvania. In over fifty years of practice Constantine Hering built up the whole fabric of homoeopathic medicine across America and made important contributions to our knowledge of homoeopathy.

He became a distinguished author, including his book entitled *Analytical Repertory of the Mind* and the condensed *Materia Medica*. His book, the *Homoeopathic Domestic Physician*, was subsequently published in no less than twenty-nine editions in seven languages. His major work was *The Guiding Symptoms*, published in 1879. It runs to ten volumes and is still used by many homoeopaths today. Dr Hering also introduced his *Laws of the Direction of Cure*, that is that cure proceeds from the above downwards, from within outwards and from important organs to lesser organs, and symptoms are cured in the reverse order of their appearance (see Chapter 5).

Constantine Hering was working on the fourth volume of *The Guiding Symptoms* when he suffered an acute heart attack. He died on

23 July 1880 in Philadelphia and was laid to rest in Laurel Hill Cemetery. The funeral was attended by a large number of relatives and friends and homoeopathic physicians, many of whom had travelled from far afield. In his book of the life of Hering, Calvin Knerr wrote 'as the dull thud of mother earth was heard shutting away from mortal sight the remains of the departed, relatives and friends slowly and sadly wended their way homeward'. Many memorial services were held throughout the United States and also in Italy and many other countries. Among the obituaries published around the world was this: 'his works will live after him. Coming generations will profit by them and like the present will honour his memory'. Dr Lippe wrote: 'one of our greatest men has passed away – I feel that he has left a record behind him worthy of emulation'.

James Tyler Kent – Leading Homoeopathy into the Modern Age

If Dr Constantine Hering was the architect of American homoeopathy then Dr James Tyler Kent was the towering intellect. It was he who, early in the twentieth century, guided homoeopathy into its modern interpretation.

James Tyler Kent was born in the town of Woodhull in New York in 1849, the son of Stephen Kent and his wife Caroline. His early education was at Franklin Academy in Pittsburgh and his higher education in Madison University, near New York.

He gained his Bachelor of Philosophy degree in 1868 and he was subsequently educated in medicine at the Eclectic Medical Institute in Cincinnati, gaining his MD in 1871.

He began his professional career in St Louis, Missouri as a physician of the eclectic (subscribing to no particular medical philosophy) school. During this time he was involved in writing for eclectic journals and he took a part in the councils of the Eclectic National College in St Louis. Kent's first wife, Ellen, died in 1872 at the tender age of nineteen years. After her death he left his home town and settled in St Louis, where he began his professional career in 1874. About this time homoeopathy came to the attention of Dr Kent through the serious illness of his second wife. Her illness had not responded to allopathic treatment and James Kent therefore consulted every physician of reputation in St Louis, but to no avail. Ellen suffered from persistent insomnia, anaemia and weakness so that she was confined to bed for months.

Subsequently she was treated homoeopathically by an elderly physician, Dr Richard Phelan, and Dr Kent was very impressed with the success of this homoeopathic treatment. As a result he became a student of Dr Phelan whose practice was close by and he became a diligent student of Hahnemann's *Organon*. Subsequently he completely converted to the practice of homoeopathy and resigned from the Eclectic Medical Association in 1879 at the age of thirty.

Dr Kent was subsequently appointed to the Chair of Anatomy in the Homoeopathic College of Missouri in St Louis. He held this position for two years until he became Professor of Materia Medica in 1883. In 1889 he was awarded the Diploma of the College. Later he became Dean and Professor of Materia Medica in the Postgraduate School of Homoeopathics in Philadelphia and held this position until 1889.

Subsequently he was Dean and Professor of Materia Medica in the Hering Medical College in Chicago. From 1903 until 1909 he was Professor of Materia Medica at the Hahnemannian Medical College and Hospital in Chicago, Illinois.

After the death of his second wife in 1890 he immersed himself totally in his work and conducted several provings of homoeopathic remedies on himself. His homoeopathic philosophy was influenced from the very beginning on the teachings of Emanuel Swedenborg.

He later married his third wife, Clara, who was also a physician, after she had come to see him as a patient. She was converted to homoeopathy by her husband and there followed many years of constructive and creative work together. Clara assisted in the writing of his major books and his other contributions to homoeopathy. James Kent's teachings and writings were to become a major influence in twentieth-century homoeopathy.

His perception, his intelligence, his intuition and logical thought advanced our understanding of homoeopathy probably to a greater extent than any other homoeopath in the twentieth century and he is still recognized today as the great master of homoeopathy. He was a prodigious writer and had a deep knowledge of the homoeopathic *Materia Medica*. He was also a brilliant teacher and an excellent physician.

Dr Kent gathered admirers far and wide, and many physicians travelled from other countries to study with him. In Great Britain, Sir Henry Tyler, the father of Dr Margaret Tyler, set up scholarships to enable doctors to travel to America to study with the great James Tyler Kent. For example, one physician who gained one of these scholarships was Dr Borland who, in turn, introduced and trained Dr Margery Blackie, later physician to Her Majesty Queen Elizabeth II.

Kent's greatest work was the *Repertory of the Homoeopathic Materia Medica*, published in 1887. It was truly a prodigious work, involving thirty-five years of painstaking application. Although nowadays many other homoeopathic repertories are available, from Boericke's 'Pocket' Repertory to the massive Complete Repertory by Roger van Zandvoorst, Kent's Repertory is still the most widely used for the selection of homoeopathic remedies. The book has also been translated into at least six other languages.

Kent also published his 'Lectures', which he entitled *Lectures on Homoeopathic Philosophy* and the first of such books was published in 1900. In these lectures he discusses the importance of the fundamental principles of homoeopathy as laid down in Hahnemann's *Organon of Medicine*. Kent's lectures on the Materia Medica, which were given at the Postgraduate School of Homoeopathics in Philadelphia, were published in 1906. Kent's other works included his *New Homoeopathic Remedies, Clinical Cases, Aphorisms and Precepts*. These works are still of great importance to students of homoeopathy today. Kent's contribution to homoeopathy is recognized world-wide: he is seen to have moved forward the frontiers of homoeopathy and increased our understanding more than anyone else, apart from Samuel Hahnemann.

In the early part of the twentieth century Dr Kent published a series of 'drug pictures'. With the support of leading homoeopathic physicians, in particular Dr Margaret Tyler and Dr Margery Blackie in the UK, he developed his concept of constitution and constitutional prescribing in homoeopathy. This approach emphasized the holistic dimension of homoeopathy, recognizing that certain people have an affinity for a particular (constitutional) remedy. The matching constitution of the patient is manifested by each person's individual physical, mental, emotional and psychological features. (See Chapters 4 and 8).

In prescribing constitutionally Dr Kent chose higher potencies, starting at 1M – one thousand centesimal, up to CM potencies and he even mentioned at one time the use of MM potencies which most homoeopaths thought to be ridiculously high (see Chapter 3). This attracted considerable criticism and led to a division between groups of homoeopaths early in the twentieth century. In particular he was opposed by Dr Richard Hughes, a senior physician in the British Homoeopathic School, who advocated the use of low potencies prescribed on pathological symptoms only. This division did the reputations of Dr Kent and Dr Hughes no good, especially when Dr Hughes described the higher potencies prescribed by Dr Kent as 'airy nothings', while Dr Kent spoke of the low potencies such as 6X or 6C prescribed by Dr Hughes as 'near to allopathic doses'.

James Tyler Kent died in his home in Stevensville, Montana in 1916. He was in the process of writing yet another book, but he developed Bright's disease (a kidney disease) and died before its completion. Dr Kent is still seen as one of the great intellects of modern homoeopathy.

Carl Von Boenninghausen – Pioneer of Homoeopathy

Dr Carl Von Boenninghausen was another pioneer of homoeopathy. He was born in 1785 and came originally from Holland to Germany. He graduated in Law in 1806 at the Dutch University at Groningen. His belief in homoeopathy came about in 1827 when he developed tuberculosis. His health deteriorated to the point when all hope of his recovery had virtually been abandoned. He wrote a farewell letter to his friend Dr Weiner who happened to be the first homoeopathic physician practising in Rhineland and Westphalia. Dr Weiner took a detailed picture of Boenninghausen's symptoms from his letter and prescribed the remedy *Pulsatilla*. Boenninghausen immediately began to

recover and by the end of the summer of 1828 he was completely cured.

Boenninghausen became a staunch believer in homoeopathy and devoted the rest of his life to its advancement. Although he never became qualified in medicine, his fame spread across to France and to America and in 1843 King Wilhelm IV bestowed upon him the right to practise medicine. He established the Homoeopathic Society of Rhineland and Westphalia in 1848 and in 1854 the Western Medical College awarded him an honorary Diploma. He also became a Knight of the Legion of Honour in 1861, bestowed by the Emperor of France.

Boenninghausen's contribution to homoeopathy came through the close friendship he developed with Samuel Hahnemann and their correspondence from 1830 until Hahnemann's death in Paris. Hahnemann and Boenninghausen discussed homoeopathic problems and the homoeopathic *Materia Medica* with animation, and Hahnemann formed the greatest respect for Boenninghausen's views.

Boenninghausen's other contribution to homoeopathy lay in his books. His first, the *Therapeutic Pocket Book*, was published in 1846 and the English translation of his Repertory by Boericke was published in 1900. His greatest work, however, was the *Aphorisms of Hippocrates with the Glasses of a Homeopath*. Hahnemann regularly corresponded with Dr Boenninghausen and letters from Hahnemann can still be seen today. In the spring of 1831, for instance, Hahnemann wrote to Boenninghausen 'if only we had a homoeopathic hospital in Leipzig with a teacher who could instruct the students in the practice of homoeopathy'. In 1835 Hahnemann wrote to Boenninghausen of his love for his second wife Melanie and Boenninghausen participated in several provings of homoeopathic remedies.

Dr Boenninghausen was an active student of Hahnemann's *Organon* and it was his opinion that homoeopathic physicians should take the totality of symptoms into consideration, as Hahnemann had instructed (see Chapter 2). He wrote 'for totality, three factors are needed – location, sensation and modalities'. He also demanded a fourth requirement, namely the concomitant symptom. Without its inclusion he believed the symptoms remained complete. Throwing further light on the totality of symptoms, Boenninghausen wrote 'a totality of symptoms is not only the sum total of symptoms but it is in itself one grand symptom of the patient'.

In his *Repertory*, Dr Boenninghausen explained that aggravations and ameliorations are simply modalities and they should be ranked as general symptoms. Many of his contemporaries believed that Boenninghausen's Repertory was the greatest masterpiece of analysis, comparison and generalization in homoeopathic literature.

In his *Therapeutic Pocket Book* Boenninghausen distributed the elements of all symptoms into seven main parts which, taken together, constitute the grand totality of symptoms. These parts were moral and intellectual faculties, seat of the symptoms (locality), sensations and complaints, sleep and dreams, fever, modalities, and concordances. Each of these parts was subdivided into rubrics containing the names of the remedies in alphabetical order under the symptoms to which they corresponded.

Boenninghausen's *Repertory* was criticized by some homoeopaths, however, who thought that the rubrics were too scattered and too limited, and found that the cross-references were not without flaws.

Furthermore, only a limited number of medicines were covered. In spite of its limitations, however, Hahnemann held Boenninghausen's literary works in high esteem and they were the greatest influence on homoeopathic physicians before the publication of Kent's Repertory.

LATER LIFE OF SAMUEL HAHNEMANN

From 1810, when the *Organon of Medicine* was published, until 1843 the fortunes of homoeopathy were largely governed by Samuel Hahnemann's success with homoeopathic treatment, the persecution he suffered at the hands of antagonistic pharmacists and physicians, and his growing band of young physicians who were turning to homoeopathy as a real alternative to conventional medicine.

Over a period of twenty years, Samuel Hahnemann and his loyal wife Johanna and their family had moved at least twenty times – Dessau, Gommern, Leipzig, Dresden, Leipzig, Stotteritz, Georgenthal, Molschleben, Mulhausen, Pyrmont, Wolfenbuttle, Brunswick, Köningslutter, Hamburg, Altona, St Jurgen, Molne, Machern, Eilenburg, Wittenburg, Dessau and, finally, Torgau. Johanna had had to cope with the frustrated, unsettled, idiosyncratic genius that was her husband, together with raising a large family and their impoverishment. For Hahnemann's medical practices had rarely provided him with sufficient income to support himself and his large family, and when they did his insistence on preparing his own medicines and his radical writings caused him to suffer persecution from doctors and the pharmacists.

At the end of January 1811, he wrote to his friend, Councillor Becker of Gotha, 'I believe you do know that I am six miles nearer you. I was threatened to be swallowed up amidst the gigantic ramparts of Torgau and I escaped here to Leipzig.' The ramparts he mentioned in this letter were a prelude to one of the most decisive battles of the Napoleonic wars, which were to cause Hahnemann to regret his choice of the city of Leipzig since it was this city that was about to become the fulcrum of the conflict.

The cultural and academic environment of Leipzig had always appealed to Hahnemann, although during his previous visits, not least his brief stay at the University, he had not been particularly happy. He promptly applied to the Dean of the Faculty of Medicine at the University of Leipzig for an appointment as a lecturer in medicine. Subsequently he was invited to deliver his own dissertation in the Great Hall of the University and, at nearly sixty years of age, he delivered his dissertation, in Latin, to a capacity audience in a masterly style. As a result he was offered the position. He had wisely omitted any mention of homoeopathy in his dissertation.

Life in Leipzig

Hahnemann opened his courses of lectures at the beginning of the new academic year in September 1812, while practising homoeopathy at his home in Burgstrasse. For a brief period he had settled into an agreeable routine but it was soon to be shattered.

In August 1813, Napoleon set up his tents on the outskirts of Leipzig with the mightiest army he had yet commanded and it was here that he engaged the allied armies commanded by Prince Karl of Schwarzenburg in the *Battle of the Nations (Battle of Leipzig)*.

During the nights of 16, 17 and 18 October, the glow of burning villages illuminated the night sky to the north and west of the city.

The battle reached its height on 18 October and the roar of the cannons, the shouts of the soldiers and the screams of the wounded rose to a crescendo. The city gates were stormed by the allied troops and Napoleon's army was decisively defeated.

Prince Karl led a triumphant column through the streets of Leipzig. During the next few days, together with the other doctors of Leipzig, Hahnemann assisted the maimed and dying soldiers, numbering more than 70,000, who filled the military hospital which had been hastily set up in the University Church.

Polluted drinking water brought a new peril to the city with an outbreak of typhus leading to a mounting death toll. This gave Hahnemann the opportunity to establish homoeopathy as a real alternative to conventional medicine. Hahnemann treated 180 typhus patients homoeopathically and achieved remarkable success. He recorded that only two had died and thus gave the first public demonstration of the efficacy of homoeopathic therapy.

Life in Leipzig returned to normal and Hahnemann resumed his bi-weekly lectures. His habit, however, was to commence his lecture by teaching orthodox medicine and then switching violently to an attack on orthodox medicine before expounding the positive features of homoeopathy. This approach won him no friends with his fellow faculty members of the University, but it caused many young medical graduates to join him in the fight for the acceptance of homoeopathy.

The storm clouds, however, were gathering about him. Samuel Hahnemann was about to experience the most severe persecution he had suffered in his whole life. In December 1819 the pharmacists (apothecaries) of Leipzig lodged a complaint to the City Council accusing Hahnemann of infringing their rights and privileges by preparing and dispensing his own medicines.

Hahnemann presented his own defence

when the case came before the court, based on the assertion that his new system of treatment was quite different and required his personal expertise in the preparation of his medicines and, in any case, since the pharmacist charged according to the weight of ingredients, the infinitesimally small homoeopathic doses would earn them virtually nothing. The Leipzig court gave judgment against him, forbidding him to prepare his homoeopathic medicines under a penalty of 20 thalers (coinage of the time).

At this time Prince Karl of Schwarzenburg, the former commander of the allied armies at the battle of Leipzig, having suffered a stroke, approached Samuel Hahnemann, requesting him to visit his palace in Austria. Hahnemann replied that he was too busy to travel, but by this time his reputation had grown to such a stature that the Prince travelled to Leipzig to be treated.

He responded well to homoeopathic treatment initially, but the Prince soon fell back on his old drinking habits, and his own personal, orthodox physicians insisted on daily venesections and other conventional treatments, which resulted in his health deteriorating rapidly. Hahnemann finally gave up the case and four days later Prince Karl died.

The reaction by the orthodox physicians to the death of Prince Karl was as swift as it was vicious. The post-mortem was conducted by Professor Clarus, Head of Clinical Science at the University of Leipzig an opponent of homoeopathy, who claimed in his report that Hahnemann's homoeopathic treatment was harmful in that it delayed the application of what he termed 'strong measures'.

Following the death of the Prince, Hahnemann's persecutors pressed for a court decision on the matter of him dispensing his own medicines. In November of that year the court ruled that Hahnemann would be allowed to dispense his own medicines, only when he was out in the country and a long distance from the nearest town or in serious cases when imminent danger did not permit the medicines to be obtained from a pharmacy. These concessions were virtually the same as those given to every doctor at that time and for all practical purposes Hahnemann found it was impossible for him to continue to practise.

Meanwhile other homoeopathic physicians were also being persecuted. Indeed, Dr Hornburg, one of Hahnemann's original team of provers, eventually suffered a martyr's fate. His medicines were confiscated and by order of the High Court he was forced to witness, in a bizarre ceremony, his homoeopathic medicines being carried away by two beagles and buried with all due ceremony in the churchyard of St Pauls Church, Leipzig. Hornburg again appeared before the courts and in 1831 criminal proceedings were brought against him by Professor Clarus (the same Professor Clarus who opposed Hahnemann and who also caused Dr Constantine Hering to leave the University of Leipzig). He was sentenced to two months' imprisonment but died just three days after the verdict.

Attacks on Samuel Hahnemann and his new therapy began to appear regularly in articles published in the Leipzig newspapers. One particular article was written by thirteen local physicians in which they challenged Hahnemann's medical judgement in the prescribing of the remedy, *Belladonna*.

Hahnemann made a spirited reply to these accusations. He wrote: 'There stand thirteen gentlemen, colleagues of mine in this town, who are struggling hard to show the readers that they envy my reputation, such as it is, my discoveries, my writings (which they will not read) and my cures which by the grace of God I have successfully effected on patients'.

Life in Köthen

Hahnemann did not wish to live in the relatively small town of Köthen, as he much preferred the cultural and social life that the city of Leipzig gave him and his family. However, he really had no choice as the ruler of this small principality, Duke Ferdinand, gave permission for Hahnemann to practise homoeopathy there, and to prepare and dispense his own medicines himself without the assistance of the apothecaries. Furthermore, the Duke and his wife declared themselves to be his first patients.

On 5 June 1821 Hahnemann took up residence in a house in Wallstrasse in Köthen and he resumed his practice of homoeopathy. There followed, over a period of about seven years, a comparatively tranquil existence for Samuel Hahnemann. His continuing success with homoeopathic treatment rapidly began to attract attention throughout the world. In 1832 he completed his final book, *The Chronic Diseases*, and, finally, in 1835, at the age of eighty, virtually retired altogether.

Cholera Epidemic

During the winter of 1831/2, a cholera epidemic swept the world from Russia across Europe and over to the eastern shores of North America. Conventional treatment was virtually ineffective and the disease claimed several hundred thousand lives around the world. Hahnemann treated many patients suffering from cholera homoeopathically and he also gave prophylactic treatment.

His homoeopathic treatment was remarkably successful. It was reported, for example, that in the Hungarian town of Raab only six patients out of 154 treated homoeopathically died, whereas more than 50 per cent of patients died when treated allopathically.

Hahnemann also wrote an important essay at this time stressing the importance of sterilization. This was written at a time when even the existence of disease bacterium was unknown. Hahnemann proposed that the spread of disease could be limited if clothes were heated in an oven for about two hours at a temperature of at least 80°C and that a high standard of hygiene on the part of everyone, with regular baths, was essential. Only in this way, he stated, could infections be annihilated. In his article he wrote, 'Cholera infection is most probably caused by a swarm of infinitely small, living organisms murderously hostile to human life'. In making this statement, the first time the existence of a disease agent was recognized, Hahnemann was at least seventy years ahead of his time. His treatment of cholera involved the use of camphor in its early stages and the homoeopathic remedies Cuprum Metallicum, Veratrum album, Bryonia and Rhus toxicodendron.

Hahnemann's New Lease on Life

In October 1834 an event occurred which was to bring Hahnemann back from his retirement to embark upon a new career which was to have a significant influence on the development of homoeopathy world-wide.

His change in circumstances was the result of a visit to Köthen by a certain Melanie D'Hervilly. An attractive Parisienne, aged about thirty and reputedly the mistress of the first President of France following the Revolution, she visited Köthen, ostensibly seeking homoeopathic treatment by the great and celebrated Dr Samuel Hahnemann. Whatever her real intentions, the fact remains that six weeks later Melanie married Samuel Hahnemann in the front room of his home in Wallstrasse. Two weeks later they set out on the fourteen-day coach journey to Paris, leaving behind his two distraught unmarried daughters, Charlotte and Louise.

It was here that Hahnemann established (or perhaps it would have been more exact to say that Melanie established) a homoeopathic practice. The practice was situated at 1, Rue de Milan, just north of the Opera in central Paris and it was here that Samuel Hahnemann practised homoeopathy from 1835 until his death in 1843. During this time homoeopathy spread around the world, across Europe, through to Asia, across the Atlantic to the North American continent and then down to South America. Kings and princes, presidents, prominent citizens and poor people alike flocked to the door of his practice for homoeopathic treatment.

Shortly after his eighty-eighth birthday Hahnemann contracted bronchial catarrh. He died peacefully in his bed in the early hours of the morning of 2 July 1843. On 11 July he was buried in the Montmartre cemetery in a public grave. The funeral was attended only by a few servants of the household, his wife Melanie, his favourite daughter Amalie and his grandson, Leopold.

Samuel Hahnemann had fought against the corruption and ignorance of a bigoted and reactionary medical profession throughout his entire professional life. He had endured persecution and contempt for seeking a more humane and natural treatment.

HAHNEMANN'S DESCENDANTS

Leopold Suss-Hahnemann, who attended his grandfather's funeral, was the only son of Hahnemann's daughter Amalie (1789–1881). Leopold subsequently emigrated to England after qualifying in medicine at the University of Leipzig, and he practised homoeopathy in London until his retirement, when he settled on the Isle of Wight. He died in 1914, leaving a daughter Amalia.

William Tankard-Hahnemann is the great, great, great grandson of Samuel Hahnemann. He served as a captain with the British army during the Second World War and is a Freeman of the City of London. He lives with his wife Elizabeth in Sussex, England and they have several grandchildren. William Tankard-Hahnemann is the patron of the British Institute of Homoeopathy and works unstintingly for the advancement of homoeopathy.

Re-Interment of Hahnemann

In March 1898, the body of Samuel Hahnemann was exhumed from his grave in Montmartre cemetery and, in the presence of representatives of homoeopathy throughout the world, his body was borne across Paris to the Père Lachaise cemetery. There, with pomp and ceremony and many speeches, his body was lowered into its last resting place. His grave is now surrounded by those of the kings and queens of France, the great generals of France, the composers Rossini and Donizetti, scientist Gay Lussac and all the great and famous of France.

Two years later, largely through the generosity of American homoeopathic physicians, a 14-ft high monument in Scottish granite was erected over the grave. It bore the inscription '*Hahnemann, fondateur de L'Homeoepathie*'. Some time later another inscription was added: *Non inutilis vixi* (I have not lived in vain).

ROYAL SUPPORT FOR HOMOEOPATHY

Until 1981 it was generally supposed that Queen Mary, the consort of King George V of England, introduced homoeopathy into the

British Royal family. However, my researches have revealed that it was actually Queen Adelaide, formerly Princess Adelaide of Saxe-Coburg-Meiningen, who was not only the first supporter of homoeopathy in England but was also probably the first person to be treated homoeopathically in England.

On her arrival in the country to marry King William IV in 1835, she was surprised to learn that homoeopathy was practically unheard of in England. On becoming ill she promptly summoned her family homoeopathic physician, Dr Stapf, from his practice in Germany. A life-long friend of Samuel Hahnemann, he travelled to England to treat the Queen in Windsor Castle. On his return home he stayed in Paris with Samuel Hahnemann where they discussed the progress of homoeopathy in England and Dr Stapf's treatment of the Queen.

Queen Adelaide had been treated by homoeopathy all her life, as an aunt of Prince Albert of Saxe-Coburg-Gotha, the second son of Duke Ernst, who was Hahnemann's benefactor when he ran the lunatic asylum in Gotha.

In 1840, Prince Albert came from Germany to marry Queen Victoria and thus renewed Royal support for homoeopathy. He arrived in England not only with the Christmas tree, but also with a box of homoeopathic medicines. Subsequently the entire royal family were treated by homoeopathy. Queen Victoria's uncle Leopold, who became King Leopold I of Belgium, was also treated homoeopathically.

Royal patronage of homoeopathy spans six generations, including King Edward VII, George V and Queen Mary, King Edward VIII, who invariably carried his homoeopathic medicines in powder doses in his pocket, and his brother King George VI, who, having been treated by the homoeopathic remedy *Hypericum* for a crushed finger, was so impressed that he named his classic-winning racehorse Hypericum after the remedy.

Her Majesty the Queen Mother has been treated homoeopathically for her entire life, like her daughter, Her Majesty Queen Elizabeth II. The Queen rarely undertakes any Royal tour without taking a box of homoeopathic medicines with her for first aid treatment. Undoubtedly the support of the Royal family has had a significant influence on the support for homoeopathy generally, not only in the UK, but also around the world. It has often been stated by those people introduced to homoeopathy for the first time, 'If it is good enough for the Queen, then it is good enough for me'.

Homoeopathy in the Twentieth Century

In the early twentieth century homoeopathy had reached a zenith, only surpassed by its support in the present day. Practised in almost every country in the world it is estimated that more than four hundred million people were receiving homoeopathic treatment. In many countries homoeopathy had become the established system of treatment for many renowned and influential people, including British Prime Minister Benjamin Disraeli; poet Robert Browning; authors Mark Twain, William Makepeace Thackeray and Charles Dickens; American President Theodore Roosevelt, John D. Rockefeller; and artist Edouard Monet.

Homoeopathic dispensaries were established in every major town in the UK and some became homoeopathic hospitals, notably those in London (Royal London Homoeopathic Hospital), Bristol, Liverpool, Glasgow, Manchester and Tunbridge Wells.

In America there were twenty-two homoeopathic medical schools and nearly a hundred hospitals where homoeopathy was practised exclusively. About one in four physicians practised homoeopathy and homoeopathic pharmacies had been established in every major city, the first being William Boericke in Philadelphia in 1835.

Factors Causing the Decline of Homoeopathy, 1920–80

During the first few decades of the century homoeopathy suffered a serious decline for a number of reasons. Allopathic medicine, with its so-called wonder drugs, in response to the public demand for an 'instant cure', had virtually swept the board when contrasted with the seemingly less spectacular homoeopathy.

1. The 'miracle drug revolution'

The so-called miracle drug revolution began in 1909 with the discovery by the German bacteriologist, Paul Ehrlich, of the synthetic arsenic compound *Salvarsan* – the first anti-bacterial drug. Its success in the treatment of syphilis, even before the discovery of antibiotics, resulted in drug companies throughout the world embarking upon a massive programme of research to develop new wonder drugs which promised instant cure.

In Britain the discovery of *sulphathiazole* proved to be the first of a new range of sulphonamide drugs. The life of Winston Churchill was saved, when he suffered from pneumonia during the Second World War, by the British discovery of the sulpha-drug M&B693. The use of amphetamines and barbiturates followed and the first antibiotic, penicillin, was discovered by Alexander Fleming in his laboratory in Paddington, London in 1928. The therapeutic activity of penicillin was developed by Professors Florey and Chain at the University of Oxford in 1938. The success of these new drugs led

physicians to believe that every disease known to humankind over the centuries would eventually be eradicated.

The drug companies were pouring millions of dollars into research and development for new pharmaceutical products.

2. Lack of homoeopathic research

Homoeopaths relied solely on the teachings of Hahnemann and the application of classical homoeopathy, but like any other scientific and medical discipline homoeopathy needed to renew itself through continuing the search for new remedies by carrying out provings and trying to determine the mechanism of cure.

3. Lack of money

Whereas the conventional pharmaceutical industry had ample funds available in which to carry out research, homoeopathy has never had a large manufacturing industry, such is the nature of the relatively simple preparation of the remedies. This disparity inevitably contributed to the stagnation of homoeopathy in the early twentieth century.

4. Internal strife in homoeopathy

Dr Richard Hughes in England rejected Hahnemann's Psora theory and his metaphysical ideas, and the teachings of Dr James Tyler-Kent in America gave pre-eminence to constitutional prescribing, whereby it was believed that certain remedies have a special affinity for certain types of people and vice versa (see Chapter 6). The disagreement between these physicians and their supporters led to a serious schism in homoeopathy. This brought about a loss of confidence in homoeopathy in general and gave the allopaths the opportunity to pour scorn on homoeopathic practice.

5. Lack of training facilities

Homoeopathy has never been included on the syllabuses of university medical schools, which has become a reason in itself for generations of medical students to consider homoeopathy to be unimportant.

Factors Leading to the Revival of Homoeopathy: 1980 to the Present Day

The tide was to turn in the early 1980s in favour of homoeopathy. Currently, homoeopathy has never had greater support, when more and more physicians recognizing the mechanistic, impersonal approach of allopathic medicine, with all its attendant hazards, have turned to the compassionate, gentle, safe and effective alternative.

1. Side-effects of modern drugs

Most people are now well aware of the potentially serious side-effects of many modern drugs. There have been many cases, over the last twenty years, of drugs being taken off the market or their supply being severely restricted because of these problematic side-effects, which are collectively termed *iatrogenic diseases* by allopaths. Homoeopathy, on the other hand, has been proved to be completely safe with no unwanted side-effects.

2. Drug addiction

The addictive nature of many doctor-prescribed drugs is now becoming clear. Patients may suffer withdrawal symptoms similar to those experienced by hallucinogenic drug users.

3. Resistance to modern drugs

The over-use and abuse of many modern drugs has led to increasing resistance by disease organisms to them. Certain antibiotics, including penicillin and tetracycline, are now required in larger or multiple doses, or in combination with other antibiotics, to effect the original therapeutic action of a single dose.

4. New, unconquered diseases

The disease virus has proved to be a very versatile organism. The confident forecast that every disease known to humanity would be conquered by the new miracle drugs has now been tempered by the realization that no real cure has yet been found for diseases such as AIDS, and many forms of cancer and heart disease.

5. Increasing health consciousness

People today are far more health conscious than in previous generations, as shown by their preparedness to seek treatment by homoeopathy and other complementary therapies, and the growth in popularity of health food stores. Another feature is the growing demand by the public for natural foods and medicines, rather than synthetic drugs.

6. The 'Green' movement

There has been growing interest over the years from sections of the public in protecting the environment, the avoidance of all forms of pollution, eating organically produced food, free of insecticides etc., and the rejection of genetically modified (GM) foods. In 1999 there were over 1,250 'organic' farms in the UK.

7. Backlash against use of animals in drug research

Anti-vivisectionists and members of animal protection societies reject the use of animals in medical research. Homoeopathy, of course, does not require the use of animals – only healthy people – in its provings.

8. Desire for personalized treatment

Many people are no longer prepared to be treated as 'disease bearers' or 'cases'. They demand that they be recognized not simply as a list of symptoms requiring a mechanistic prescription, but to be treated as people. A common complaint heard is, 'The doctor did not even look at me. He just scribbled out a prescription'. The desire to be treated as a unique human being is consistent with the personalized, holistic approach of homoeopathy.

9. Cost of modern drugs

The massive drugs bill of the National Health Service has become an increasing burden over the years, and many treatments are now out of the reach of many people because of their excessive cost. Natural homoeopathic medicines, prescribed in minute doses, are available at a fraction of the cost of allopathic drugs.

10. Demonstrable success of homoeopathic treatment

Computer databases have, in recent years, built up case studies demonstrating the remarkable efficacy of homoeopathic treatment in both acute and chronic diseases. Homoeopathy has now been practised for nearly two hundred years. It is safe, free from unwanted side-effects, non-addictive, inexpensive and effective.

It will be pertinent to close this chapter by reproducing a statement made by Dr Pemberton Dudley during the ceremony when Samuel Hahnemann's body was finally placed in the Père Lachaise cemetery in Paris in 1898, since it encapsulates the whole ethos of homoeopathy:

Whatever estimate science may finally place on the discovery and doctrines of Samuel Hahnemann, his personality and his work have achieved a position which must render them perpetually historic. His teachings have been so interwoven in the entire fabric of medical progress, that neither the wear and tear of time, nor the dissections of criticism will ever be able to disassociate them. Hahnemann's teachings are destined inevitably to run through the texture of every page in the future annals of medicine. Hahnemann's position is more than merely transitional. He proclaims both an epoch an era. He represents both discovery and progress.

OPPOSITION TO HOMOEOPATHY

It is important that students of homoeopathy know the history of homoeopathy and understand why the medical establishment was so opposed to it, as most of these factors are just as relevant today. These factors also help us to understand the whole ethos of homoeopathy, as well as to anticipate and be prepared to rebuff ill-founded criticism.

Homoeopathy is an intrinsically safe, humane and compassionate therapy, with massive clinical evidence to support its therapeutic efficacy, so why should it arouse such, sometimes hysterical, opposition?

1. Conventional medical practice was rooted in tradition and monolithic. It had undergone no fundamental change for

centuries and the innovation stirred up a fierce loyalty to the status quo.

2. The teaching of medicine was based on a rigid conformity with accepted practice.

3. Homoeopathy was not – and for the most part it is still not – included in any university syllabus. This was a reason in itself for young medical graduates to reject homoeopathy.

4. Hahnemann's somewhat dogmatic and inflexible attitude, together with his sensitivity to criticism, inculcated hostility to homoeopathy by the physicians. The acceptance of homoeopathy would have been greater had Hahnemann not continued his own attacks on allopathic medicine.

5. Professional jealousy was exhibited by allopathic physicians who did not enjoy the professional status they have today. A code of ethics was non-existent at that time.

6 The allopathic physicians simply could not understand a compassionate approach when the physician–patient relationship of that time was based on fear and intimidation. Medicines had to be foul tasting to be effective and the treatment of the mentally ill involved restraint and brutal chastisement.

7. Having been trained in the administration of massive material doses of drugs, the allopaths could not accept that the infinitesimally small homoeopathic doses employed could possibly be effective. 'The little fist of homoeopathy shakes the giant of disease?'

When it was proven even later that high potencies of homoeopathic remedies theoretically contained no molecules of the ' active ingredients' of the mother tincture (see Chapter 3), their credulity was stretched even further.

8. Opposition by the apothecaries was based largely on mercenary considerations The small homoeopathic doses threatened their income, which was based on the quantity of drugs they dispensed. They did not know how to prepare the new homoeopathic remedies anyway.

9. In a climate of quackery and charlatans claiming new elixirs, the physicians were naturally suspicious of the integrity of any new therapeutic claims.

QUESTIONS

Answers are given on page 187

1. Samuel Hahnemann carried out his first epoch-making experiment with the drug:

- -

2. Samuel Hahnemann gained his medical degree in the year:

1810　　　　**1796**　　　　**1779**　　　　**1821**

3. Medicine in the eighteenth and nineteenth centuries was based largely on techniques:

- -

4. Samuel Hahnemann introduced his new system of medicine in the book entitled:

- -

5. Testing the effect of natural substances on healthy people is called

a. -

6. Constantine Hering proved the remedies

- -

7. Kent's philosophy was influenced by the teachings of.

- -

8. Hahnemann demonstrated the effectiveness of homoeopathy after the Battle of Leipzig in his treatment of

- -

9. Hahnemann's final resting place in Paris is at

- -

10. Side-effects of allopathic drugs are termed

- disease.

CHAPTER 2
Basic Principles and Philosophy of Homoeopathy

Law of Similars. Law of the Infinitesimal Dose. Homoeopathy as an holistic therapy. Artificial disease. Complex disease. Totality of symptoms. Vital force. Stimulation of the body's natural defence (immune) mechanism. Classical homoeopathy.

ORIGINS

It could be said that homoeopathy is as old as medicine itself. The 'father of medicine', Hippocrates, stated in around 400BC, 'By similar things a disease is produced and through the application of the like, it is cured'. Thus, he stated in a simple way the basic principle of homoeopathy.

Around 350BC, Aristotle wrote, 'Often the simile acts upon the simile'. Again he was touching upon the basic homoeopathic principle, the treatment of like with like. And Galen, the Greek physician who practised in Rome around AD150, wrote of 'natural cure by the likes'.

Paracelsus, the medieval Swiss physician, philosopher and medical reformer, wrote around 1500, 'Sames must be cured by sames'. Paracelsus was not quite in tune here in that in homoeopathy we are concerned with similars (homoios) and not sames (homos), nor opposites as in conventional medicine (hetero).

THE FIRST PRINCIPLE OF HOMOEOPATHIC MEDICINE

A German physician Dr George Stahl wrote the first accurate definition of the fundamental principle of homoeopathy in 1623: '**To treat with opposite acting remedies is the reverse of what it ought to be. I am convinced that disease will yield to, and be cured by, remedies that produce similar affections**'.

Accurate as he was in defining what came to be known as the Law of Similars, like all those philosophers before him, Dr Stahl did not put the principle to the test. It was left to Dr Samuel Hahnemann to develop the theory and apply it to clinical practice. Thus it was Hahnemann who was to become known as the father of modern homoeopathic medicine.

We learned in Chapter 1 of Samuel Hahnemann's epoch-making experiment with the remedy *Cinchona*. It will be recalled that he wrote at that time, 'Peruvian (Cinchona) bark which is used as a remedy for intermittent fever (malaria) acts because it can produce symptoms similar to those of intermittent fever in healthy people'. In his *Organon of Medicine*, published in 1810, which is considered to be the year of birth of modern homoeopathy, Hahnemann expressed it thus, '**Every medicine which,** among the symptoms it can cause in a healthy body, reproduces those most present in a given disease, capable of curing that disease in the swiftest, most thorough, and enduring fashion.'

This is the Similimum principle, or the Law of Similars. By this principle a homoeopathic remedy is selected for its ability to produce similar symptoms in a healthy person to the disease symptoms experienced by the patient.

The word itself was derived by Hahnemann from the Greek words *homoios*, meaning like or similar, and *pathos*, meaning suffering or disease. Hence the literal meaning of the word homoeopathy is 'like (or similar) suffering' or 'like (or similar) disease'. The word encompasses, therefore, the basic principle of homoeopathy, that of treating like with like.

Hahnemann wrote, '*Similiar similibus curentur*' or 'Let likes be treated by likes'. He had asserted the truth of the homoeopathic principle in this Latin phrase. At the same time he attacked the allopathic physicians who wrote of 'homopathy', claiming that by using the spelling 'homo' (same), they clearly did not understand the basic principle of homoeopathy.

Hahnemann also coined the word 'allopathy' to describe conventional or orthodox medicine, from the Greek words *allo*, meaning other, and *pathos*, meaning suffering or disease, hence, rather dismissively, 'other therapy'.

The Immunization Principle

It is significant that Samuel Hahnemann first wrote the word 'homoeopathy' in an article he wrote in 1796. In the same year Dr Edward Jenner, who practised in Gloucestershire, England, had inoculated a young boy with cowpox to protect him against the more serious disease, smallpox,

and thus demonstrated the principle of immunization for the first time. The idea of immunization had been considered by Hahnemann, but he did not take it up because of the risk involved. If we consider the principle of immunization – -similar symptoms of a milder disease to protect a person against a more serious disease – we must ask ourselves, is this the same principle? *Similia similibus*?

It was a remarkable coincidence since they did not know of one another, that Hahnemann introduced homoeopathy in the same year as Jenner introduced immunization, as the close relationship between the two therapies is now clearly understood. It is also significant that Edward Jenner suffered the ridicule of his reactionary medical colleagues, as did Samuel Hahnemann.

The Law of Similars

In his article published in 1796, entitled 'Essay on a New Principle for Ascertaining the Curative Power of Drugs and Some Examinations of Previous Principles', published in Hufeland's Journal – the same article in which he first used the word homoeopathy – Hahnemann wrote:

One should proceed as rationally as possible by experiments of the medicines on the human body. Only by this means can the true nature, the real effect of the medicinal substance be discovered. Every effective remedy incites in the human body an illness peculiar to itself. One should imitate nature which at times heals a chronic disease by an additional one. One should apply in the disease to be healed, particularly with a chronic disease, that remedy which is liable to stimulate another artificially produced disease as similar as possible, and the former will be healed – *Similia Similibus* – like with like. In order to cure disease, we must seek medicines that can excite similar symptoms in the healthy human body.

Hahnemann's basic philosophy of medicine was summarized in the first two aphorisms (or paragraphs) in his *Organon of Medicine*. In paragraph 1, he wrote, 'The physician's highest calling, his only calling, is to make sick people healthy to heal, as it is termed'. Not for Hahnemann the cruelty and the barbarity of the medicine of his contemporaries, not for him the deliberate delay in making the sick healthy in order to accumulate higher fees; he simply wanted to heal.

In paragraph 2 of the *Organon* he wrote, 'The highest ideal of therapy is to restore health rapidly, gently, permanently; to remove and destroy the whole disease in the shortest, surest, least harmful way according to clearly comprehensive principles'. The latter phrase emphasized the fact that his new therapy – homoeopathy – was based on clear principles as opposed to the empirical nature of conventional medicine.

Hahnemann went on to explain the action of the basic homoeopathic principle of the Law of Similars. In paragraph 29, he wrote, 'In homoeopathic cure this vital principle which has been dynamically untuned by natural disease is taken over by a similar and somewhat stronger artificial disease through the administration of a potentized medicine that has been accurately chosen for the similarity of its symptoms. Consequently the weaker natural disease is extinguished and disappears. From then on it no longer exists for the vital principle which is controlled and is occupied only by the stronger artificial disease. Thus delivered it can again maintain the organism in health'.

Hahnemann declared the Law of Similars as the basic law of therapeutics. The great

American homoeopathic physician Herbert Roberts observed that there can be no general consideration of the Law of Similars unless it comprises consideration of symptoms as one of the necessary elements. Comprehension of the symptoms of a given case was one of the primary factors and only insofar as one comprehends the expression of disease in these phenomena is one equipped to follow the Law of Cure in any particular case. Symptoms are the only representative expression of the diseased state. This includes sensations as expressed by the patient, appearances in all parts of the body, the varied circumstances under which these symptoms were recorded, and the varied groupings of these symptoms in any consideration of the case.

When a symptom is noted under certain circumstances and not under others, Roberts explained, this obvious relation between the symptom and its related circumstance is in itself a symptom, or rather a part of a symptom, the sensation being quite incomplete without the expressed relationship of circumstance.

Two or more symptoms may appear together, or synchronize with each other, so frequently that they are really one symptom and must be considered as such in the practitioner's analysis. As nothing in nature can be represented by a single property, so no disease can be represented by a single symptom.

No medicine can cure any disease unless it acts on all the disease parts, either directly or indirectly, thus the more similar symptoms of a drug resemblance to the disease, the nearer is its vital approach to the disease and the more dynamic its action.

No medicine can effect a perfect cure unless it has a curative action on every diseased part and in just the proportion that each part manifests the disorder.

Homoeopathic medicine administered according to the Law of Similars is the true regulator of the vital energy, that vital essence that is synonomous to the patient him or herself.

The Law of Similars is therefore as fundamental as any law in nature . As Roberts described it, it is a law of universal adapt-ability to human sickness.

TOTALITY OF SYMPTOMS

In paragraph 34 of the *Organon*, Hahnemann wrote:

> 'The artificial disease brought on by the homoeopathic medicine does not only have to be stronger in order to cure the natural disease, but above all it must have the greatest possible similarity of symptoms to the natural disease being treated.' Thus, the two sets of similar symptoms mutually destroy one another since they cannot co-exist in the organism. He then said, 'Two dissimilar diseases can co-exist if they occur simultaneously which is termed a complex disease. In this case, one disease is suspended whilst the other runs its course.'

Further he wrote:

> The only infallible guide in the art of healing [homoeopathy] teaches us in all provings [tests] conscientiously conducted, that the medicine that produced upon a healthy human body the greatest number of symptoms similar to those of the disease being treated is the only one that will cure. Administered properly this medicine will rapidly, thoroughly and permanently destroy the totality of the symptoms of the disease, which means the whole disease itself.

Hahnemann had already stressed the importance of the totality of symptoms in every individual case of disease. In paragraph 7 he wrote:

> It is the totality of symptoms, the outer image expressing the inner essence of the disease that is of the disturbed 'vital force' that must be the main, even the only means by which the disease allows us to find the necessary remedy. The only one that can decide the appropriate choice. In every individual case of disease the totality of symptoms must be the physician's principal concern.

Therefore it is clear that only the closest possible match will ensure the selection of the correct homoeopathic remedy according to the principle of the Law of Similars. Unless the practitioner determines all the presenting symptoms of the patient then it is not possible to accurately choose the remedy with the optimum curative effect. Otherwise the practitioner may well be left with the choice of several remedies of apparently equal potential therapeutic effect. However, Hahnemann made it clear that rarely would one find a remedy with 'proving symptoms' that were an exact match.

Continuing with paragraph 7 Hahnemann wrote, 'A single symptom is no more the whole disease than a single foot is a whole man'. Thus again he stressed the importance of determining all the symptoms to describe the whole disease. He explained, however, that an exact comparison is rarely achieved between the symptoms of the natural disease and the proving symptoms of the chosen homoeopathic remedy.

Kent emphasized Hahnemann's teaching thus, 'The removal of the totality of the symptoms is actually the removal of the cause. The totality of symptoms is a broad thing. If it's the essential of the disease. It is all that enables the physician to individualize between diseases and between remedies.'

The conventional view is that symptoms are a direct manifestation of a disease, whereas by the homoeopathic principle it is believed that the symptoms are a manifestation of the fight to overcome the disease by the body's natural defence mechanism.

Homoeopathy, therefore, seeks to stimulate the symptoms of the natural disease, however briefly, and not to suppress them as is generally the case in allopathic treatment. By stimulating the symptoms homoeopathic medicine assists the body's natural immune system and brings about a cure by natural means. The adage 'helping the body to help itself' is appropriate in this context.

THE LAW OF THE INFINITESIMAL DOSE

Paracelsus (1527) first mooted the principle when he wrote, 'It depends on the dose whether a substance heals or becomes a poison. The dose must be very small' Even at this time, he recognized that 'a good poison can make a good remedy'.

Hahnemann's old adversary, Professor Clarus, Head of Clinical Science at the University of Leipzig, publicly stated that the 'little fist' of homoeopathy only delayed the application of 'strong measures'. Like most of his contemporaries he believed that the infinitesimally small homoeopathic doses employed in homoeopathy could not compare in therapeutic efficacy with the massive macrodoses of allopathic medicines.

Having developed a range of homoeopathic medicines by carrying out provings on healthy people, Hahnemann needed to establish the minimum dose consistent with its therapeutic efficacy when

the toxic nature of the remedy had been eliminated. He found to his surprise that not only were the infinitesimally small doses he achieved by serially diluting the remedy no longer toxic with no side-effects, but they also retained their therapeutic effectiveness. Further dilution of the remedy followed by succussion (see Chapter 3) actually enhanced or modified the therapeutic action!

For most of the twentieth century the organic substance, *phenolphthalein*, was prescribed by allopathic physicians world-wide as a laxative. The impure brown powder that was manufactured was indeed an effective remedy. At the time I was working as a research scientist and was given the task of purifying the substance by serial recrystallizations in a solvent to confirm the belief that the pure substance would be even more efficacious than the impure product.

To my surprise the perfect, colourless crystals of pure phenolphthalein I produced proved to have a lesser therapeutic effect than the impure material. It was concluded that there must be an impurity which had been discarded in the purification process that was even more effective as a laxative.

Attempts to extract and isolate this 'wonder' impurity failed, since the quantity present in the original impure phenolphthalein was very, very small -on the scale of a homoeopathic dose. Thus, here is an example where the allopaths believe that a massive dose of this drug is essential, when homoeopaths know that only an infinitesimally small dose of an impurity is necessary!

For centuries the principle of the minimum dose, or less means better, had been mooted. The French physician Maupericius succinctly defined the principle in the eighteenth century thus, 'The quantity of action necessary to effect any change in nature is the least possible. According to this principle the decisive amount is always a minimum – an infinitesimal amount.'

VALIDATION OF THE LAW OF THE INFINITESIMAL DOSE

Hugo Schultz, Professor of Pharmacology at the University of Griswald, and Rudolf Arndt conducted a research programme using yeast growth to validate the claim of the efficacy of the minimum dose.

The **Arndt–Schultz Law** states that small doses of drugs encourage life activity, large doses of drugs impede life activity, and very large doses of drug destroy life activity. Thus, we can say that the efficacy of the drug is inversely proportional to the dose.

Dr Karl Kotschau in Germany in 1926 repeated the work of Arndt and Schultz and provided scientific validation of what became known as the **Law of the Infinitesimal Dose**. The results are presented as a biphasic response curve (or time response curve). (See diagram below).

Very low dose – curve A: results in a controlled stimulation, followed by a gradual return to normal. This would represent the homoeopathic dose.

Moderate dose of drug – curve B: stimulates to a greater extent, followed by inhibition and then a return to normal. This is the fundamental cycle of action and reaction that is common to any stable energy system.

Too large a dose – curve C: produces a very sharp stimulation initially, followed by a steep drop into the potentially lethal inhibiting range, culminating with the lethal dose limit, LD100.

We are reminded that the definition of a catalyst in chemistry is a very small quantity of a substance that can bring about a large amount of chemical change. This is consistent with the homoeopathic view that the infinitesimally small (catalytic) dose stimulates or catalyses the body's immune system. Conversely, a catalytic poison is defined as a large quantity of a substance that

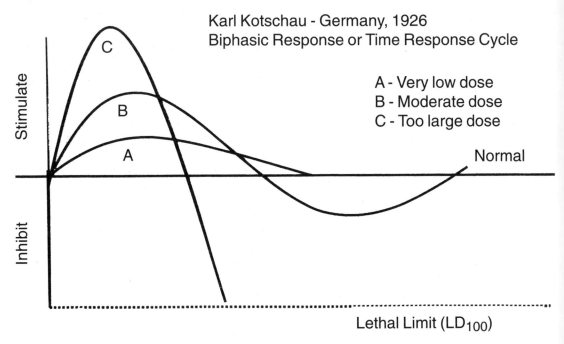

Karl Kotschau - Germany, 1926
Biphasic Response or Time Response Cycle

A - Very low dose
B - Moderate dose
C - Too large dose

Normal

Lethal Limit (LD$_{100}$)

can reduce or destroy a chemical reaction (allopathic).

In 1955, Wilder developed his *Law of Initial Values* that underlined the difficulty in establishing a minimum dose. Whereas the Arndt–Schultz Law was based on the pharmacological dose, Wilder expressed his rule in terms of the varying sensitivity of different organisms to a given dose level. What is a small dose for one individual may be a medium dose for another and a large dose for yet another, yielding different effects in each individual.

THE VITAL FORCE

Hahnemann was not the first to postulate the existence of a 'life-force' that motivates the living organism. Others who have put forward similar theories include the physicist, Isaac Newton, who described this force or energy as the subtle spirit; Luigi Galvini, the inventor, who wrote of the life-field; the British biochemist, Rupert Sheldrake, who spoke of morphogenic fields; and the Swedish cancer expert, Bjorn Nordestrom who described it in terms of biological closed circuitry. Since ancient times practitioners of Chinese acupuncture have recognized this force and call it Chi, while the Hindus call it Prana.

In the *Organon of Medicine*, Hahnemann wrote:

In the state of health the spirit-like vital force (or dynamis) animating the material human organism reigns in supreme sovereignty. It maintains the sensations and activities of all the parts of the living organism in a harmony that obliges wonderment. The reasoning spirit who inhabits the organism can thus freely use this healthy living instrument to reach the lofty goal of human existence. (paragraph 9).

In the following paragraph, Hahnemann wrote, 'Without the vital force, the material organism is unable to feel or act or maintain itself. Only because of the material being the vital force that animates it in health and disease can it feel and maintain its vital functions. Without the vital force the body dies.'

Paragraph 11 of the *Organon* tells us:

When the man falls ill it is at first only this self sustaining spirit like vital force everywhere present in the organism which is untuned by the dynamic influence of the hostile disease agent. It is only this vital force, thus untuned, which brings about in the organism this disagreeable sensations and abnormal functions that we call disease.

Homoeopathic treatment restores the balance, harmony or equilibrium of these forces and effects the cure.

Bio-energy or the vital force is essentially an holistic phenomenon. It embraces the whole person in mind, body and spirit. In the healthy person these bio-energetic forces are in balanced harmony. In disease the forces become weak; there is a loss of harmony and equilibrium; and there is an imbalance in the normal, stable, vibrational state.

Thus homoeopathy aims to restore the harmonious, balanced energy waves of the vital force in the healthy condition from the disturbed, unbalanced energy pattern of the diseased condition. Homoeopathic medicines achieve this by stimulating the body's natural defence mechanism or immune system with infinitely small homoeopathic doses.

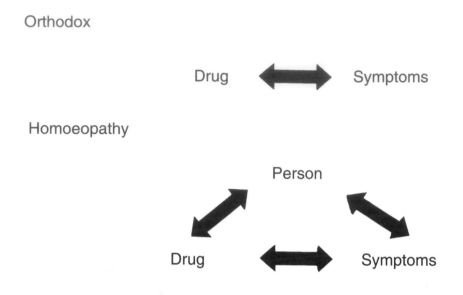

The Holistic approach of Homoeopathy

In paragraph 11 of his work the *Organon of Medicine* Hahnemann wrote:

The smallest dose of a properly potentized medicine [see Chapter 3] in which calculation shows that there is only an infinitesimal amount of material substance left, so little that it cannot be imagined or conceived, exerts far more healing power than strong material doses of the same medicine. This very subtle dose which contains almost none of the original active ingredient but the spirit-like vital medicinal force released and freed can bring about, solely by its dynamic power, results that are impossible to obtain with crude medicinal substances even in massive doses. The specific invisible medicinal force of these highly potentized remedies does not depend on their physical surfaces. On the contrary it is the invisible energy of the crude substance released and freed which is to be found in the minute impregnated globule or its solution. Upon contact with living tissue this medicinal force acts dynamically on the whole organism.

Hahnemann continued, 'It is only the pathologically untuned vital force that causes diseases. The whole pathological disturbance of the dynamis reveals the whole disease.'

In paragraph 15 Hahnemann wrote:

In the invisible interior of the body the suffering of the pathologically untuned spirit like dynamis or vital force, animating the organism and the totality of the perceptible symptoms that result and that represent the disease are one and the same. The organism is the material instrument of life but it is no more conceivable without the life-giving regulating vital force or dynamis – the two are one.

In paragraph 17 he wrote, repeating the philosophy he gave in paragraph 1 of the *Organon*:

A cure is the elimination of all the perceptible signs and symptoms of disease. Consequently the physician has only to eliminate the totality of the symptoms in order to remove the pathological instrument of the vital force thereby entirely removing and enabling the disease itself. When the disease is destroyed then health is restored and this is the highest goal, the only goal of the physician who knows the significance of his calling.

The wisdom of Hahnemann's philosophy is still appropriate today, although we would now seek to explain the nature of vital force in terms of the neuro-immuno-endocrine system of the body and the action of homoeopathic remedies on these systems.

THE HOLISTIC THIRD PRINCIPLE OF HOMOEOPATHY

In his book, *The Chronic Diseases; Their Peculiar Nature and Their Homoeopathic Cure*, Hahnemann wrote:

The physician's first duty is to enquire into the whole condition of the patient, the cause of the disease, his/her mode of life, the nature of his/her mind, the tone or character of his/her sentiments, his/her physical constitution and then especially the symptoms of the disease.

Thus Hahnemann signalled that, in taking a case, the physician must look beyond the presenting symptoms.

Homoeopathy is termed an holistic medical practice in that it treats the whole person (sometimes 'holistic' is spelled 'wholistic' which is probably more appropriate in this context). Homoeopathy recognizes that every person is unique and, as the late Dr Margery Blackie said, 'It is the patient not the cure'.

The causative factors of an illness are of prime importance in the homoeopathic system, since they enable practitioners to optimize the individualistic approach to treatment. Thus, homoeopathy seeks to treat the whole person and not simply the disease symptoms. (See Allergens chapter 9).

The allopathic physician Dr Pietroni wrote (1984):

Although the quality of the individual parts must influence the illness, the biochemical model cannot take into account the social, psychological and environmental context in which the parts function, how the person thinks, behaves and relates to others or where life-style influences the ways parts operate. We should replace the mechanistic approach to the study of health and disease with a humanistic approach where sharing, caring, loving, touching and hoping play an important role in our endeavours to treat the patient. The holistic approach to medicine as practised in homoeopathy recognizes that the whole person is more than the sum of their parts. The whole person is multi-dimensional, responding to a particular social environment. Mind and body constantly interact with one and other, thus the homoeopathic practitioner must be concerned with biological, psychological, emotional and social factors since holistic medicine accepts that all these systems influence one and another.

The psychological state of the patient is therefore of great importance in deciding the homoeopathic treatment. Many illnesses result from the patient's lifestyle with all its excesses. Conventional medicine is often concerned simply with suppression of the severity of symptoms, which suggests to the patient that they are getting better, and this then in turn encourages them to continue the habits and lifestyle that were the cause of the disease in the first place.

Patients receiving homoeopathic treatment should not be passive; they must be prepared to avoid excesses and eradicate circumstances in their lives that cause them agitation, depression and stress. The removal of these will stimulate the body's natural defence mechanism, thereby increasing the efficacy of the homoeopathic remedy. Patients must be prepared to change their lifestyle, their habits, their diet and perhaps their control of stress. The homoeopathic practitioner needs to develop the empathy, the patience and the understanding needed to encourage the patient to mobilize their own healing potential.

The additional dimension of the 'person' complicates homoeopathic practice enormously, but at the same time it enriches homoeopathy as a humane therapy.

Robin Logan in *The Homoeopathic Treatment of Eczema* (Beaconsfield) has

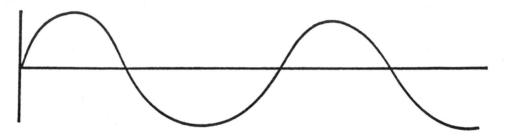

Harmonious, balanced energy waves (vital force) in the healthy condition

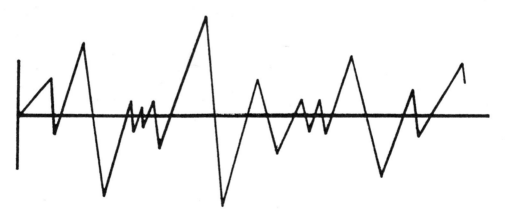

Disturbed, unbalanced energy pattern in diseased state

clarified the classical definition of holism:

Holistic medicine should mean more than 'treating everything'. It does not simply infer the application of a separate therapy, as is the case in homoeopathy, a different remedy for each individual complaint. Nor is it sufficient to define holism as an approach that addresses the mind, body and spirit of the person. In the deepest sense it is more than merely a form of humane all encompassing medicine. To understand homoeopathy, when practised as its founder, Samuel Hahnemann, originally intended is to understand the true meaning of holism. That is we recognize the need to heal the mind, body and spirit and pay attention to all the patient's symptoms, but additionally perceive the inter-relatedness of all aspects of the person and seek to make connections between seemingly disparate signs and symptoms. By maintaining an open mind and a broad perspective and by applying our inherently holistic therapy, we can exemplify holism it its most profound expression.

SUMMARY OF THE THREE BASIC PRINCIPLES

Thus, we have the three basic principles of homoeopathy: the Law of Similars; the Law of the Infinitesimal Dose; and its holistic nature. Of these principles, the Law of Similars, based on Samuel Hahnemann's inspiration, is fundamental and immutable. It is the basis for classical homoeopathy.

In the foreword to Steven Decker's definitive translation of Hahnemann's *Organon of the Medical Art*, Jeremy Sherr has written, 'Becoming a homoeopath does not depend on the study of the Materia Medica. It is not defined by prescribing potentized remedies, nor is it reliant on remembering the Repertory. It is the living and understanding of these laws which endows our medical practice with true healing.'

Below is a summary of the main features of homoeopathic medicine that distinguish it from orthodox treatment:

1. Homoeopathy does not suppress symptoms, but cures naturally
2. It does not seek to diagnose and name a disease, but only requires a knowledge of the totality of symptoms of the disease.
3. There are no unwanted side-effects. The remedies are completely safe.
4. The remedies are non-addictive.
5. No animal experiments are necessary nor desired (only healthy people can participate in provings).
6. Individualized treatment of the whole patient is undertaken.
7. Homoeopathy cures naturally, safely and gently by stimulating the body's natural immune system.
8. Infinitesimally small doses are prescribed (potencies, see Chapter 3).
9. Remedies are prescribed following the application of the Law of Similars –the fundamental precept of homoeopathy laid down by Samuel Hahnemann.

QUESTIONS

Answers are given on page 187

1. The literal meaning of the word 'homoeopathy' is:

----

2. The similar, but stronger symptoms induced in the organism by the homoeopathic remedy are called the disease.

----

3. The literal meaning of the word 'allopathy' is:

----

4. The Law of the Minimum dose is defined by the

----

5. Two dissimilar diseases which can occur simultaneously in the organism are termed

a. ---

6. The 'vital force' was also given the name by Hahnemann.

----

7. Disease-like symptoms induced by giving natural substances to healthy people are called

----

8. The equilibrium or balance of the _____ is restored by homoeopathic treatment

----

9. The principle of immunization was introduced by

----

10. State two other names used to describe the 'vital force':

CHAPTER 3

Sources and Preparation of Homoeopathic Remedies

Homoeopathic Pharmacopoeias. Plant, animal, mineral and biological sources. Mother tinctures. Potentization. Succussion. Potency series. Dilutions. Potency equivalents. Trituration. Medication. Pharmaceutical forms. Quality control.

HOMOEOPATHIC PHARMACOPOEIAS

All homoeopathic remedies are prepared in compliance with the procedures laid down in the Homoeopathic Pharmacopoeia, and in accordance with the principles and teaching of Samuel Hahnemann. The quality standards adopted are relatively uniform in the Homoeopathic Pharmacopoeias published throughout the world.

The first edition of the British Homoeopathic Pharmacopoeia (BHomP) was published as early as 1876 and 1882, but surprisingly the second edition was not published until 1994. This edition, published by the British Homoeopathic Manufacturers Association, includes the Bach Flower Remedies which are not strictly homoeopathic. It is based on the English translation of the German Homoeopathic Pharmacopoeia first published in 1825.

The French Homoeopathic Pharmacopoeia was published in 1965 and a new edition was published in 1983. It is a comprehensive reference work and has full legal status in France. The Indian Homoeopathic Pharmacopoeia was published in 1991 in four volumes.

The Homoeopathic Pharmacopoeia of the United States (HPUS) was published in eight editions between 1895 and 1979. The current, ninth edition was produced by the Homoeopathic Pharmacopoeia Convention of the United States (HPCUS), which was established in 1980. Part I of the Pharmacopoeia which covers, *inter alia*, General Pharmacy and Criteria for Eligibility was published in 1989. Part II consists of several hundred monographs of fully proven – and therefore approved – homoeopathic remedies. Further monographs are being added from time to time.

HOMOEOPATHIC MANUFACTURING LEGISLATION

The manufacture, packaging, labelling, sale and supply of all homoeopathic remedies in the UK is controlled by the same legislation that applies to allopathic medicines, that is the Medicines Acts 1968 and 1971, under which all medicines **bearing a medicinal claim on their labels** require a product licence (PL) issued by the Medicines Control Agency (MCA).

Procedures for the manufacture and labelling of homoeopathic medicines under the Medicines Act must conform with what is described as Current Good Manufacturing Practice (CGMP) and their quality is at least as high as their allopathic counterparts.

'Non-orthodox practitioners' (NOP), which includes homoeopathic practitioners, may be granted mixing and assembly licences by the MCA to cover local dispensing activities.

SOURCES OF HOMOEOPATHIC REMEDIES

Every natural substance on planet Earth that is capable of inducing disease-like systems in the healthy person is potentially a homoeopathic remedy. Currently, however, there are about 3,000 homoeopathic remedies available world-wide, including allergens (see Chapter 5).

The sources of homoeopathic remedies may be classified as follows:

1. Plants – including shrubs, vegetables, flowering plants and trees, bulbs or corms, berries, fruits, seeds, buds and young shoots.
2. Animals – including insects, spiders and sea creatures.
3. Minerals – including the elements and mineral salts.
4. Biological – Biological remedies are sub-divided between nosodes, isodes and sarcodes.

Plant Remedies

Plant sources represent the largest group and account for over 60 per cent of all homoeopathic remedies. The part or parts of plant material to be taken for the preparation of homoeopathic remedies are laid down in the Homoeopathic Pharmacopoeias. The parts may be the whole plant, including flowers and the roots, or parts of a plant such as the roots alone, the fruit, the berries, the leaves or the bark of a tree.

Non-resinous barks of trees are collected from young trees in the late autumn, while barks from resinous trees are collected during the development of the leaves and blossom. Berries and fruits are gathered when they are ripe, as perfect specimens. Seeds are often dried and stored in laboratories for future use. Bulbs and corms are lifted from the soil in March and April when they are beginning to grow. In some cases buds and young shoots of plants (so-called gemmotherapy, see Chapter 9), which are rich in growth factors, such as minerals, vitamins, hormones, auxins, flavenoids and gibberelins, are used.

Plant specimens are best collected in dry, sunny weather and are carefully inspected for insects, moulds and other imperfections before shaking in distilled water to remove dirt.

All plant material is grown in organic nurseries without the use of pesticides, fertilizers etc. Although the analysis of plant material varies appreciably when grown in different countries or different areas, due to variations in the soil composition in which they grow, research has shown that it has little effect on their therapeutic efficacy. Some examples of plant remedies are as follows (see also Chapter 8 for more detail):

ALLIUM CEPA.: Prepared from whole fresh bulb gathered in July and August prior to the growth of the rhizome in the second year.
CAULOPHYLLUM: The blue cohosh, also known as yellow ginseng, is the source of this remedy. The roots and rhizomes are used.
CINCHONA OFFICINALIS (China): Commonly known as Peruvian bark or the

Quina Quina tree. The dried, yellow bark of the tree is used. This remedy, of course, was that used in Hahnemann's epoch-making experiment (see Chapter 1).

COLCHICUM AUTUMNALE: The corm of the autumn crocus, as it is commonly called, is used when lifted in the early autumn. The corm is characterized by its main constituent, a poisonous substance called colchicine.

DROSERA ROTUNDIFOLIA: Commonly known as sundew. The whole flowering plant is used for the remedy.

LYCOPODIUM CLAVATUM: This remedy is prepared from the crushed spores of the shrub, commonly known as clubmoss. The spores are pale yellow and form a very mobile powder.

NUX VOMICA: The dried seeds of the five orange berries contained in the fruit of the poison nut tree which grows in northern Australia are used. The seeds, which have a high strychnine content, are very poisonous. The remedy is fully titled Strychnos nux vomica.

RIBES NIGRUM: The remedy is prepared from the buds of the blackcurrant bush gathered in the early spring.

SYMPHYTUM OFFICINALIS: This remedy, commonly known as comfrey or knitbone, is prepared from the fresh root of this herb.

Animal Remedies

Homoeopathic medicines derived from animals include marine animals, snakes and insects. With the exception of the honey bee and scorpion, the remedy recently proved by the well-known British homoeopath Jeremy Sherr, dead animals are used. They are usually crushed and dried before use. Almost 20 per cent of all homoeopathic remedies are derived from animals.

APIS MELLIFICA: The remedy is prepared from the whole, live honey bee.

BUFO RANA: The remedy is prepared from the dried venom of the very poisonous toad, Bufo vulgaris.

SEPIA OFFICINALIS: This remedy is prepared from the brown inky juice of the cuttlefish or squid, which is released from a sac beneath its mouth on the approach of a predator. This brown pigment has been used by artists for centuries.

TARENTULA HISPANIA: The whole of the Spanish spider or Lycosa tarentula is used in the preparation of the remedy.

Mineral Remedies

Mineral remedies are divided into two categories:

1. Those which are soluble in alcohol/water and those which are insoluble in alcohol/water. Mother tinctures of insoluble minerals are prepared by a process known as trituration (see later in this chapter).
2. Simple elements or mineral salts.

Some examples of mineral remedies are as follows:

CALCAREA CARBONICA: This remedy, commonly known as calcium carbonate, might have been classified as an animal remedy, as it is derived from the soft, middle layer of the oyster shell. It contains small quantities of impurities such as magnesium carbonate, but it is believed that these impurities enhance its therapeutic effectiveness. In view of its source, the remedy is sometimes called *Calcarea carbonica ostrearum*.

ALUMINA: Commonly known as aluminium hydroxide of the formula $AL(OH)_3$ in its powdered form.

AURUM METALLICUM: The bright yellow metal is used in its powdered form to prepare the remedy by trituration (see later in this chapter).

FERRUM PHOSPHORICUM: Commonly known as iron phosphate. This remedy consists of a mixture of hydrated ferrous phosphate, ferric phosphate and oxides of iron.

MAGNESIUM PHOSPHORICUM

Commonly named magnesium phosphate or phosphate of magnesia, the remedy is prepared from the hydrated crystalline form of this mineral salt.

PHOSPHOROUS: This remedy is prepared from the element in its yellow *allotropic* form.

Biological Remedies

Biological remedies fall into three main categories: nosodes, isodes and sarcodes. Approximately 10 per cent of homoeopathic remedies are from biological sources.

Nosodes

Nosodes are the most important category. They are prepared from human diseased tissue, for example pus, and their action in homoeopathy is profound. Examples of nosodes are Psorinum, Medorrhinum, Influenzinum, Tuberculinum and Syphilinum (Lueticum) (see Chapters 4 and 8). Nosode remedies have the suffix '*inum*'.

Isodes

Isodes are prepared from diseased or healthy tissue taken from the patient him or herself for use by that patient only. They are therefore a highly individualized form of homoeopathic medicines. Examples are blood, hair or skin.

Sarcodes

Sarcodes are derived from the healthy glands, organs or tissues of animals, usually slaughtered animals such as cattle, sheep or pigs. They are used in the branch of homoeopathic medicine known as organotherapy. Examples of sarcodes are thyroid glands, hypothalamus, liver, kidney, lung or heart (see Chapter 9).

Homoeopathic Remedies from Unclassified Sources

This category includes a wide range of remedies including allergens, for example mixed grass pollen, dog hair, cat hair or feathers, Electricit (produced with an electric current), x-ray, Sol (from sunshine) and Lunar (from moonlight).

More than a hundred remedies are prepared from allopathic drugs. These remedies are used largely to counter the side-effects of these drugs (iatrogenic) or therapeutic withdrawal.

PREPARATION OF HOMOEOPATHIC REMEDIES

There are three stages in the preparation of homoeopathic remedies, as follows:

Stage 1. The preparation of mother tinctures
Stage 2. Potentization
Stage 3. Medication

Stages 1 and 2 are combined when preparing potencies of insoluble minerals or elements (trituration). The medication, Stage 3, simply involves the preparation of the remedy in a pharmaceutical form which is convenient for administration to the patient.

Preparation of Mother Tinctures

Mother tinctures are produced either as clear liquids or as solids in the triturated form. The liquids range in colour from colourless to a pale straw through yellow, dark yellow, green, yellow/green, brown or dark red. Mother tinctures are denoted by the Greek letter *phi*. Mother tinctures are abbreviated to MT (TM in France), for example, Sepia MT.

Step A – Maceration

Maceration of the plant, animal, mineral or biological material is achieved by comminution followed by squeezing plant material or grinding in a 'liquidizer'. The mincing or 'mulching' of the plant material squeezes out the juice (succus) of the plant. Succulent plants harvested in full flower, such as Calendula officinalis (marigold), produce about 350ml of succus or juice per kilogram of the plant material. The resulting solution is filtered. The final tincture represents about one-tenth of the concentration of the original drug.

Step B – Extraction

The macerated material is extracted with a solution of ethyl alcohol (ethanol) and distilled or de-ionized water. The amount of alcohol is varied according to the water content of the starting material. For example, a succulent plant, which may contain as much as 80 per cent of its weight as water, will require a relatively high quantity of alcohol. On the other hand, a relatively dry starting material, such as the bark of a tree, will require a low concentration of alcohol and a high quantity of water. Thus, the strength of alcohol in mother tinctures may vary between 33 and 88 per cent (volume/volume).

Step C – Ageing process

The 'mulch' thus produced, consisting of the suspension of the undissolved macerated material in the juice or solvent, is allowed to stand in a well-stoppered amber glass container in a cool, dark place. Ageing periods may vary from one hour or up to one month with occasional stirring or shaking of the contents before the final stage.

Step D – Filtration

The final step in the preparation of the mother tincture is to separate the solid material from the liquid. Filtration may be by gravity using a filter cloth or paper, pressure or vacuum. The bright, clear liquid filtrate is the mother tincture.

It is essential that the mother tincture remains clear. Any sediment that may form on ageing must be filtered. If the clear solution becomes very cloudy on ageing then it must be re-filtered or rejected. Cloudiness often arises by precipitation of dissolved material through loss of alcohol evaporating via a loosely-fitting stopper.

Preparation of Potencies

This essential process, which is unique to homoeopathy, is sometimes also called dynamization.

There are three main methods of potentization: Hahnemannian, Korsakovian and the Skinner method. The classical method of potentization was devised by Samuel Hahnemann. Today it is still the principal method and it is usually carried out by hand.

Potentization converts mother tinctures into homoeopathic potencies by a strict scientific procedure. Hahnemann developed his method following years of experimentation. It is carried out in two distinct stages – dilution followed by succussion. The potentization cycle is shown in the diagram.

Potentization involves the sequential or serial dilution of the mother tincture with mixtures of 20 per cent ethanol/distilled water or 30 per cent ethanol/distilled water (volume/volume). Each dilution

Potentization Cycle

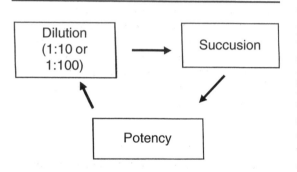

step is followed by the process termed succussion by Hahnemann (literal translation: to shake violently). Succussion involves vigorous shaking of the diluted tincture with an impact on a hard, resilient surface. The succussion is thought to energize the resulting potency. Hahnemann's writings showed that he placed increasing import-ance on the succussion step: in the first edition of the *Organon of Medicine* he instructed that there should be ten impacts; in the second to fifth editions he instructed at least ten impacts; and finally in the sixth edition he instructed one hundred impacts, which is the number employed today.

Attenuation

The use of the word attenuation to denote potency, dilution or the process of potentization in many textbooks is not entirely appropriate and confuses some students. The Homoeopathic Pharmacopoeia of the United States, 8th edition (now superseded), defined potencies in the following way: 'Standard scales of attenuation contains just as much of the drug substance as the preceding attenuation'.

An attenuated substance cannot be described as potency since dilution alone, without succussion, does not produce a potency. The standard dictionaries of the UK, Canada and United States define attenuation as to make thin in consistency, to separate particles of a substance, to weaken in force, to lessen in value or degree or to make less dense. None of these definitions suggest that attenuation is the correct word in the context of potencies and potentization. Another word, *fluxion*, which is sometimes used in older textbooks, is best consigned to history.

Potency Series

There are four series of potencies, namely:

1. Decimal series
2. Centesimal series
3. Millesimal series
4. LM series

Let us consider the preparation of each of these series of potencies.

Decimal Series of Potencies

The decimal series of potencies are based on serial or sequential dilutions in the ratio of one to ten. That is, one part of mother tincture to nine parts of 20 per cent or 30 per cent alcohol/water, producing an overall dilution of the original starting material of 1:10. Thus, the method of preparation of a decimal potency is as follows:

To 1ml of mother tincture in a glass vial is added 9ml of the alcohol/water solution. The mixture is then succussed by striking the vial one hundred times on a hard resilient surface, such as a leather-bound book or a rubber pad. This produces the first decimal potency which is written 1X.

To 1ml of the 1X potency thus produced in a new clean container is added 9ml of the alcohol/water solution. The diluted potency is then succussed as before, producing the second decimal potency, that is a potency of 2X.

1ml of the liquid potency 2X is then diluted further by repeating the procedure above to produce a potency of 3X and so on up the decimal series – 4X, 5X, 6X, 7X etc.

Summarizing, we have the first decimal potency (1X), which represents a dilution of the original mother tincture of one part in ten parts (1:10) (10^{-1}); 2X represents the second decimal potency and represents a dilution of the original mother tincture of 1:100 (10^{-2}); 3X is a dilution of one part mother tincture in one thousand parts of alcohol/water, 1:1000 (10^{-3}) and so on.

This process of serial dilutions and succussions is normally repeated up to a maximum of two hundred times to produce a liquid with a decimal potency of 200X.

Centesimal Potencies

The centesimal potencies are prepared in exactly the same way as the decimal series of potencies, but here a dilution ratio of 1:100 rather than 1:10 is employed. Thus the procedure is as follows:

To 1ml of mother tincture in a glass vial, 99ml of alcohol/water (20 per cent or 30 per cent alcohol) solution is added. The mixture

is then succussed one hundred times to produce the first centesimal potency of 1C.

To 1ml of the liquid potency 1C produced in the previous step, a further 99ml of alcohol/water is added. The mixture is again succussed one hundred times to produce a potency of 2C, that is the second centesimal potency.

The process may be repeated to produce centesimal potencies of 3C, 4C, 5C and so on. In practice, centesimal potencies are prepared up to 100,000C, which is normally abbreviated to CM.

Summarizing, we have the first centesimal potency 1C, which represents a dilution of the original mother tincture of one part in one hundred parts (1:100) (10^{-2}); 2C represents the second centesimal potency with a dilution of the original mother tincture of one part in ten thousand parts (1:10,000) (10^{-4}) and so on.

Millesimal Series of Potencies

In the early part of the twentieth century the millesimal series of potencies was introduced, based on serial or sequential dilutions in the ratio of 1:1000. However, this series never proved popular and is now rarely, if ever, used today.

Potencies are prepared by sequential or serial dilutions starting with 1ml of the mother tincture diluted with 999ml of alcohol/water solution to produce the first millesimal potency.

Millesimal potencies are denoted by 1m, 2m, 3m, 4m etc. and sometimes 1mm, 2mm, 3mm, 4mm etc. (note: 1M = 1,000C).

LM Series of Potencies

Shortly before his death in 1843, Samuel Hahnemann wrote in his diary, 'I have just completed the sixth edition of my *Organon*

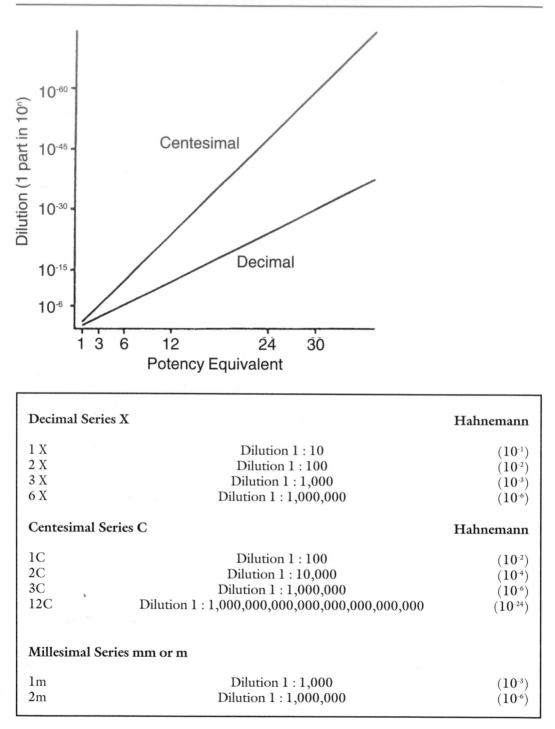

of Medicine and it is nearly the most perfect of all'. After his death homoeopathic physicians approached his wife Melanie, requesting a copy of the manuscript. However, in spite of offers of large sums of money, particularly by American homoeopathic physicians, Melanie refused to part with it. The manuscript was eventually lost after Melanie's death and it was not published until 1921 after William Boericke found the manuscript in Paris.

To the consternation of the homoeopaths, Hahnemann had introduced a totally new series of potencies with a different method for their preparation. The first five editions of his Organon all instructed the preparation and prescription of decimal and centesimal potencies, but in this sixth edition he introduced the so-called fifty millesimal series or the LM series of potencies.

The delay in the publication of the sixth edition of the Organon of Medicine thus fundamentally changed the practice of homoeopathy. Homoeopaths had become accustomed to preparing and prescribing decimal and centesimal potencies over more than seventy years, and all their experience was related to these series of potencies. They were therefore reluctant to change to the new LM potencies. Some homoeopaths even suggested that Hahnemann was becoming senile when he wrote the sixth edition and it should not be taken seriously. Certainly there were a few anomalies in the text which strengthened this view and, of course, Hahnemann was not alive to answer questions himself. Had the sixth edition of the Organon been published when it was written there is no doubt that students of homoeopathy would now be taught to use LM potencies, and the decimal and centesimal potencies would have been a matter of history! As it is centesimal and decimal potencies have remained the preferred series and, until only recently, LM potencies have remained untried.

LM potencies are based on serial or sequential dilutions of a liquid potency of 3C (the third centesimal potency) in the ratio of one part to fifty thousand parts of alcohol/water. The procedure is as follows:

One grain (0.06g) of the third centesimal potency (3C) in powder form is dissolved in 500 drops (30ml) of pure water, giving a dilution of 1:500.

1ml of solution is diluted again with 99ml of alcohol (94.9 per cent or 95 per cent volume/volume) to fill the vial to approximately two-thirds of its volume. According to Hahnemann this volume is ideal for the succussion process which follows.

The vial is succussed one hundred times. This produces a medicating potency of LM1 (the first LM or fifty millesimal potency).

One drop of the LM1 medicating potency is added to 500 granules, each granule weighing 0.0006g. Thus one granule absorbs 1/500 of a drop of the medicating potency.

One of these granules is then placed in a new, clean vial and dissolved in one drop of water. Ninety-nine drops of 94.9 per cent/95 per cent ethyl alcohol are added to the vial.

The liquid is then succussed one hundred times to produce a potency of LM2.

The process is repeated to produce successively LM3, LM4, LM5 and so on to a maximum of LM30 (the thirtieth LM or fifty millesimal potency).

Hahnemann wrote in the Organon, 'My new method of potentization to produce LM potencies produces medicines of the highest power and the mildest action'.

The advantages of LM potencies are that they work as deeply and as powerfully as the higher decimal and centesimal potencies but, as Hahnemann pointed out (Organon, paragraph 70), LM potencies have a more

LM Potencies

First LM Potency	LM1	0/1	(5c)*
Second LM Potency	LM2	0/2	(7.5c)
Third LM Potency	LM3	0/3	(10c)
Fourth LM Potency	LM4	0/4	(12.5c)**
Fifth LM Potency	LM5	0/5	(15c)
etc., etc.			
Thirtieth LM Potency (maximum)	LM30	0/30	(73c)

*Each LM step represents a rise in dilution equivalent on centisimal scale of 2.5c
**Avogadro Limit (12c)

Summary of Potency Series		
Series	Symbol	Dilution Ratio
Decimal	X	1:10
Centesimal	C	1:100
Millesimal	m	1:1,000
LM	LM1	1:50,000
(Fifty Millesimal)		

gentle action without significant aggravations. If an aggravation does occur, it will do so towards the end of the treatment rather than at the beginning, as with decimal and centesimal potencies. Furthermore, the procedure whereby the LM potency is progressively increased, starting with LM1 at the beginning of the treatment and then progressing up to a maximum of LM30, is a simpler procedure than with treatment by decimal and centesimal potencies.

The use of LM potencies and other potency series will be discussed in more detail in Chapter 5.

Korsakovian Potentization

General Simeon Korsakov, a Russian General in the Army of Czar Nicholas, was a keen homoeopath. In 1832 he proposed a new method of potentization. Surprisingly, Hahnemann declared that his new method was 'both judicious and useful' and it was widely adopted.

Basically Korsakov's method followed the Hahnemann technique exactly, except that while the Hahnemann method required a new, clean vial for each potentization step, Korsakov proposed that the same vial be used for each step. He claimed that if one chose carefully the dimensions of the vial, when the vial was inverted 1ml of the solution remained adhering to the internal walls of the vial. Thus the vial could then be returned to its upright position and would be ready for further dilution and succussion in the next potentization step.

Clearly this method was advantageous in that it was much faster than the Hahnemannian method and, of course, it economized on the numbers of vials used. Hand succussion by the Hahnemannian method for high potencies was very time consuming and nowadays, in practice, potencies above 200X or 200C are normally prepared by the Korsakovian method.

Another advantage of the Korsakovian method is that it lends itself easily to automation and computerization, which can be used to speed up the potentization process even more.

A disadvantage of the Korsakov method is that variations in ambient temperature and pressure in the laboratory affect the viscosity and surface tension of the potency liquid in the vial, causing the quantity of the liquid adhering to the internal walls to vary. With the Hahnemann method the scientific procedure ensures total accuracy.

Korsakov potencies are sometimes written, for example, 6K, 30K, 200K and so on. Alternatively, they may be written 6CK, 12CK, 200CK etc. To differentiate the two procedures, Hahnemannian potencies are sometimes written 6CH, 30CH, 200CH, etc.

Skinner Method of Potentization

Another potentization method is used principally by the Boericke and Tafel company in Philadelphia, United States. The method devised by Dr Skinner is in fact a combination of the Hahnemannian and Korsakovian methods of potentization. The potentization is carried out by a 'dynamizer'. Basically Skinner's method involves the use of the Hahnemannian procedure up to a

Comparison of Potentization Methods

Method	Advantages	Disadvantages
Hahnemannian	Scientific	Labour consuming
	Accurate	Slow
		Uses many vials
Korsakov	Faster	Not so accurate
	Less labour used	
	Easily automated	
	or computerized	

potency of 30C or 30X, followed by the Korsakov procedure for higher potencies up to CM (100,000C).

Very high potencies up to CM, or even MM, are prepared by the Skinner method using continuous 'fluxion' whereby a continuous flow of water is run into a glass vial containing 5ml of the starting centesimal potency over periods of up to several days.

Trituration

Insoluble minerals or metals that will not dissolve in alcohol/water solutions require potentization in the solid form by the process known as *trituration*. The object is to reduce the substance to the finest possible powder and, at the same time, to energize it. The process of trituration is to reduce the crystals or powder of the starting substance, which will not dissolve in the standard alcohol/water solution used in liquid potencies, to a degree of fineness that will permit their solubilization.

The procedure is as follows: 1g of the insoluble substance is ground to a fine powder and placed in a mortar. 1g of pure lactose powder is then added to the mortar and the mixture is stirred for a few minutes, after which the lining of the mortar is scraped with a spatula to remove any particles adhering to the sides. The mixture is rubbed with the pestle for a total of four minutes. A further 3g of pure lactose is then added and the process of rubbing and stirring is repeated. Finally, 5g of pure lactose is added and the process of rubbing and stirring is repeated. The resultant finely divided mixture represents the first centesimal triturated potency, that is a **solid potency** of 1X.

The trituration–potentization process is then repeated using 1g of the first decimal triturate and adding a further 9g of pure lactose in aliquot quantities as described above. The rubbing and mixing procedure is then repeated to produce the second solid centesimal potency by this trituration process.

It is believed that the heat energy generated by the grinding of the two powders together provides the equivalent energy of 'succussions' to the solid potency thus produced.

The trituration process is both time-consuming and requires much energy on the part of the pharmacist. Therefore, this solid potentization method is switched to the more convenient liquid potentization as early as possible. In practice the changeover is carried out when a triturated potency of 7X is reached. Thus at this point 1g of the solid triturated potency of 7X is dissolved in 9ml of 20 per cent or 30 per cent ethanol/water solution and the mixture is succussed one hundred times. This produces a liquid potency of 8X. At this potency level the original insoluble starting mineral or metal is sufficiently diluted to be within the solubility co-efficient of the alcohol/water solution. Thereafter the normal standard liquid potentization process may be employed through 9X, 10X, 11X, 12X and so on.

Solid triturated potencies may be compressed directly into so-called soft tablets and they may then be administered to the patient as a remedy.

Examples of triturated remedies are Calcarea carbonica (calcium carbonate), Hepar sulphuris (calcium sulphide), Aurum metallicum (gold metal) and Plumbum metallicum (lead metal).

Medication

The medication stage in the preparation of homoeopathic remedies is simply the conversion of the liquid homoeopathic potency into a pharmaceutical form suitable for administration to the patient.

Liquids

In this case the liquid potency produced in the normal manner in a 20 per cent or 30 per cent volume/volume concentration of ethanol/water may be given orally to the patient without further processing. Sometimes mother tinctures may be given orally, for example Crataegus (for angina pectoris).

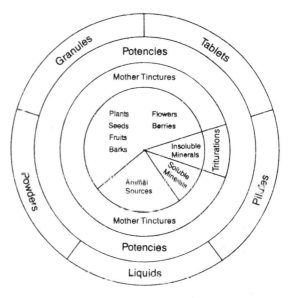

The mother tincture is sometimes taken with water. Liquid potencies are transferred to dropper bottles of the type using a plastic insert in the neck of the bottle or fitted with the conventional rubber bulb. Dropper bottles are usually of amber glass and are available in 5ml, 10ml, 20ml, 30ml, 50ml or 100ml capacities.

Solid Forms

(a) Powders
Lactose powder is impregnated with the liquid medicating potency. Medicating potencies are prepared using 95 per cent ethanol in the final dilution stage of the potentization process. For example, to prepare a medicating potency of 30C, 1ml of

Abbreviations and Symbols	
phi	Mother tincture
TM	Mother tincture
MT	Mother tincture
Tinc	Tincture
C	Centesimal potency
X	Decimal potency
H	Hahnemann or Hahnemannian
K	Korsakovian
CH	Centesimal potency prepared by Hahnemann method
CK	Centesimal potency prepared by Korsakov method
CS	Centesimal potency prepared by Skinner method
M	1,000
L	50
LM	50,000
N	Potency number
D	Decimal potency (France)
Hom	Homoeopathy or Homoeopathic
DHPh	Diploma in Homoeopathic Pharmacy
RPh	Registered Pharmacist
BHomP	British Homoeopathic Pharmacopeia
HPUS	Homoeopathic Pharmacopeia of United States
Trit.	Triturate
b.i.d.	Twice daily
t.i.d.	Three times daily
q.i.d	Four times daily

a 29C potency (20 per cent or 30 per cent alcohol) is diluted with 99ml of pure alcohol. The mixture is then succussed one hundred times to produce a medicating potency of 30C. This medicating potency may then be used to impregnate various solid dose forms, such as powders or tablets.

The use of medicating potencies is necessary because high concentrations of water tend to dissolve the sugar base used and cause the powders, tablets or pills to partially dissolve and coagulate.

Powders may be given individually and they are particularly useful when the treatment involves the use of a placebo dose. The powders are individually numbered and the patient is instructed to take the powders in numerical order. Thus some doses will consist of pure lactose only.

(b) Tablets

Homoeopathic tablets are available in two forms. *Soft tablets* are prepared by mixing the solid powder potency with pure lactose powder or medicating pure lactose powder with a liquid potency and then compressing the mixture into the tablet form. This process is usually done by hand and produces a soft tablet that dissolves readily in the mouth. Biochemic remedies or cell salts are usually produced in the soft tablet form.

Combining the placebo material with the therapeutic ingredient *before* compressing is a feature of the allopathic method.

Hard tablets are produced by compressing a mixture of pure lactose (80 per cent by weight) and pure sucrose (20 per cent by weight) in a conventional tabletting machine. The combination of these natural sugars has a greater binding power than lactose alone and hence a higher degree of hardness of the tablet. The hard placebo tablets thus produced are then medicated by dripping or spraying the liquid medicating potency on to the tablets.

Hard tablets are round with a diameter of approximately 4mm, double convex shape, and ten thousand tablets weigh approximately 1kg. The medication of these placebo hard tablets involves dripping or spraying the liquid medicating potency (95 per cent alcohol) on to the tablets. Two or three drops of the medicating potency are sufficient to medicate fifty hard tablets.

(c) Pills (Pillule)

In non-English speaking countries, particularly in France, pills are sometimes called granules and this can cause confusion. Nowadays tablets have largely replaced pills, as patients have become used to the former with allopathic prescriptions. Pills are prepared from pure lactose (lactose BP or USP), with a small amount of sucrose added. They are spherical in shape with a diameter of approximately 4mm and prepared in the style of confectionery. The standard dosage is two pills (or two tablets) for adults and one to two pills for children.

(d) Granules

Granules, sometimes called globules, are simply small pills. Approximately 1mm in diameter, they are often called 'poppy seed' granules. They are usually prescribed for infants or old people by application to the mouth on the tip of a clean spoon.

(e) Creams, ointments and lotions

All these pharmaceutical forms are for topical application. Ointments are prescribed to a lesser extent nowadays, as they are sticky and can stain clothes. They are usually based on soft paraffin or lanoline.

Creams are more popular and are prepared from a non-staining water base. Low potencies such as 1X, 2X, or 3X are usually employed.

Lotions are water based or simply liquid potencies (20–30 per cent alcohol/water) for one or more remedies.

Mother tinctures are quite commonly used for topical applications in their natural form or incorporated in a cream or lotion. Examples are Arnica MT for warts to Calendula MT or lotion for cuts and sores.

(f) Suppositories

Like their allopathic counterparts, homoeopathic suppositories are conical-shaped with a rounded apex. They are for rectal, urethal or vaginal use, weighing about 0.5g (for vaginal use, suppositories are more globular in shape).

The remedy is mixed with a base of glycerin, gelatin or beeswax which is melted and poured into a mould and then refrigerated. They are finally rolled in foil to prevent contamination.

QUALITY CONTROL

All manufacture of homocopathic medicines is governed in developed countries by current good manufacturing practice (CGMP) and quality control is no less stringent than in the manufacture of allopathic medicines. Thus, homoeopathic medicines are accepted by most health authorities as meeting their criteria for both safety and quality.

As Hahnemann implies, a homoeopathic practitioner, however well experienced and knowledgeable, can only be as good as the purity of the medicines.

Since he regarded the preparation of the medicines as an exact science (see Chapter 8), only a scientific system of quality control to ensure the integrity of the products is appropriate. The purchase of cheap homoeopathic remedies from doubtful sources is to be avoided.

Analysis

The analysis of constituents of homoeopathic medicines presents special problems owing to the very high dilutions involved. Even low potencies such as 6X or 6C, with a relatively high concentration of active ingredients, are barely within the accuracy of the most modern and sophisticated scientific instruments. For this reason only mother tinctures are analysed comprehensively and accurately. The normal methods employed are organoleptic tests (colour, smells, clarity etc.), separate analysis for percentage by weight, or parts per million, of each ingredient or the procedure known as thin layer chromatography (TLC).

TLC involves immersing a glass plate coated with a very thin film (up to 250 microns) of inert substance, such as powdered silica in a liquid solvent, such as a mixture of butyl alcohol and acetic acid. A spot of the mother tincture is placed at the base of the plate above the liquid level. The different migration rates of the dissolved substances in the mother tincture produces bands across the plate characteristic of each mother tincture. The more simple lighter molecules travel further up the plate than the heavier complex molecules in the mother tincture. The bands resemble a product bar code; the thicker the band the greater the quantity of the particular constituent of the mother tincture. Chromatographs of mother tinctures being tested are compared with standard plates of known mother tintures for alignment of the various bands.

Higher potencies are now tested by sophisticated nuclear magnetic resonance analysis (NMR) (see Chapter 4).

Although proper analysis of mother tinctures and potencies is essential, it must be remembered that their dilution goes beyond the accuracy of modern scientific procedures. The aim in homoeopathy is to capture the subtlety and essence of the natural substance used for the remedy.

Care of Homoeopathic Remedies

If properly prepared and stored, almost all homoeopathic remedies have an indefinite 'shelf life' and retain their therapeutic potential fully. For legal purposes, however, a nominal shelf life of five years is often stated on the label.

Liquid tinctures must always be bright and clear. Sometimes, after prolonged storage in a cool place, the clear liquid may turn cloudy or a precipitate may be deposited at the bottom of the container. In this case the mother tincture is passed through a filter to separate the solid material. The clear filtrate is then re-bottled and may be used again.

The general rules for the proper storage and care of all homoeopathic remedies are as follows:

Thin Layer Chromatography

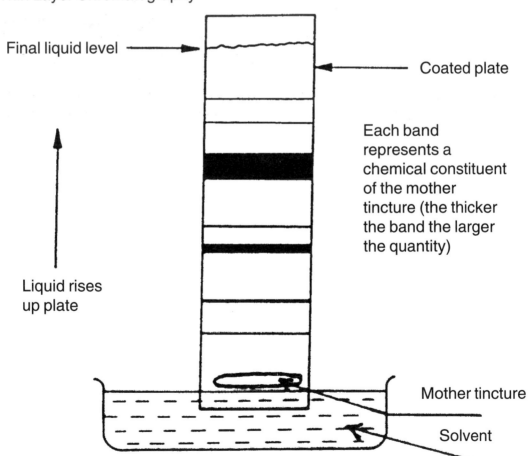

Final liquid level

Coated plate

Each band represents a chemical constituent of the mother tincture (the thicker the band the larger the quantity)

Liquid rises up plate

Mother tincture

Solvent

STORAGE OF HOMOEOPATHIC REMEDIES

1. Do not touch the solid pharmaceutical form with the hands. They are very sensitive and are easily contaminated. Solid doses may be taken orally by tipping the tablet or pills into the cap of the container and then placing on to the tongue.
2. Homoeopathic medicines, particularly liquids, are best stored in amber glass containers.
3. Storage must be in a cool/dark place such as a basement or cellar.
4. Remedies must be protected from sunlight.
5. Remedies must be kept away from strongly smelling substances, such as camphor (Hahnemann) or garlic.
6. Bottles or vials must be firmly stoppered. Loss of alcohol by evaporation through a loosely fitted stopper is probably the main cause of deterioration of a remedy.

7 Remedies must be rejected if a colour change is observed, including darkening.
8. If possible, the passage of homoeopathic medicines through electronic security checks at airports etc. should be avoided. If the medicines are kept as 'carry on' luggage, most security officers will allow them to be put to one side while the passenger passes through the 'gate', when they may be collected.
9 All containers must be properly labelled at all times and labels must not be altered.
10 All homoeopathic medicines should be obtained from licensed, reputable manufacturers who guarantee their purity and quality.

(Note: If properly stored, homoeopathic remedies will retain their therapeutic effectiveness indefinitely.)

55

QUESTIONS

Answers are given on page 187

1. State the natural source of the following remedies:

(a) Nux vomica: --

(b) Cantharis: --

(c) Rhus toxicodendron: --

(d) Sepia officinalis:--

(e) Lachesis mutus: --

(f) Plumbum metallicum:--

2. State the common English names of the following mineral remedies:

(a) Calcarea carbonica: --

(b) Hepar sulphuris: --

(c) Kalium bichromicun: --

(d) Natrum muriaticum:--

(e) Argentum nitricum: --

3. Give the names of three polycrest remedies:

(a) --

(b)--

(c) --

4. List the four potency series:

(a) --

(b) --

(c) --

(d) --

5. State the dilution ratio of the starting material for each serial (or sequential) dilution for each of the four potency series:

(a) --

(b) --

(c) --

(d)--

6. State the dilution of the original mother tincture of a potency of the following:

4X --

2C --

30X--

24C ---

7. At what dilution of the original mother tincture can we switch from preparing solid potencies of insoluble substances by trituration to preparing liquid potencies?

----

8. What is the difference between a soft and a hard tablet in homoeopathy?

----

9. Write the prefix or suffix for the potency number which denotes:

(a) Decimal potency

(b) Fifty millesimal potency

----

10. List four conditions for the proper storage of homoeopathic remedies:

(a) --

(b)--

(c) --

(d)--

CHAPTER 4
Homoeopathic Philosophy

Hahnemann's teaching. Provings. Miasms. Constitution concept. Acute and chronic diseases. High potencies: the Avogadro limit. Aggravation. Modalities. Classical homoeopathy. Suppression. Palliation. Sequential therapy. Hippocratic oath. Differential diagnosis.

MIASMS

'It will help the physician to bring about a cure', Hahnemann wrote in paragraph 5 of the *Organon*, 'if he can determine the most probably exciting cause in an acute disease and the most significant phases in the evolution of a chronic, long lasting disease, enabling him to discover its underlying cause, usually a chronic miasm'.

Hahnemann had already defined an acute disease and a chronic disease. An acute disease is of sudden onset with a definite start and finish. It is of short duration with violent but superficial symptoms. It is probably infectious. On the other hand, a chronic disease is characterized by criteria that are virtually the opposite of acute disease. The time of onset is uncertain. The symptoms are deep-seated and insidious. A chronic disease is of long duration and the patient will probably never be cured. Chronic diseases are hereditary, passed down through generations of a family.

In *The Chronic Diseases* (page 28) Hahnemann stated:

> It was a continually repeated fact that the non-venereal chronic diseases after being time and time again removed homoeopathically, always returned in a more or less varied form with new symptoms or they re-appeared annually. This gave me the first clue that the homoeopathic physician has not only to combat the well defined chronic disease but that he has always to encounter only some fragment or a more deep seated original disease. There must be an underlying cause in a chronic disease.

Thus he assumed that chronic disease lay dormant in the body and returned periodically in one form or another. He dedicated his life to the search for a therapy that would go to the root of the original disease.

Hahnemann concluded that there were three sources of chronic infections which he called miasms. The word miasm comes from the Greek word *miainein*, meaning to pollute or to defile. The choice of this word relates to the biblical concept of disease, especially skin diseases, being related to contamination or uncleanliness. It is now clear why he chose to describe the cause of the chronic disease as 'underlying' in paragraph 5 of the *Organon*.

Paragraph 78 of the *Organon* tells us that:

> The true natural chronic diseases are those that arise from a chronic miasm and that, left to themselves without their specific remedy, continue to increase indefinitely tormenting the patient with ever greater suffering to the end of his days. These diseases are by far the gravest, most numerous scourges of humanity after those caused by medical abuse. Most robust, physical constitution, the most orderly way of living and the most lively of vital energy are not equal to eradicating them.

Paragraph 79 teaches us that until now only syphilis has been somewhat recognized as a chronic miasmatic, one that, untreated, disappears only in death. Sycosis (figwort disease), similarly irradicable by the vital force when untreated, has not been recognized as a particular chronic miasmatic disease which it most certainly is. It is thought to be cured with the destruction of the outgrowths on the skin.

The miasm is defined as a taint or stigmata, either inherited or acquired, which permeates every cell in the body and is then passed on genetically to each succeeding generation. Thus certain people are predisposed to certain illnesses from the time of their birth. Hahnemann recognized that the two miasms known at that time – **sycotic** originating from gonorrhea and **syphilitic** originating from syphilis – were traceable to venereal disease, hence his choice of the name.

In paragraph 80 of the *Organon* he introduced a third miasm, which he named **psora**. Hahnemann believed that most chronic diseases have their origin in psoric or skin infections, and in functional and nervous disorders. Furthermore, he claimed that every person is exposed to the psoric miasm.

In paragraph 80 of the *Organon*, Hahnemann wrote:

> Immeasurably more widespread and consequently far more important than the two preceding miasms is the chronic miasm of psora. While the other two manifest their specific chronic inner malady by the venereal chancre and the cauliflower-like excrescencies respectively, the inner monstrous chronic miasm of psora announces itself after the complete internal infection of the entire organism through a characteristic cutaneous eruption accompanied by an unbearable tickling itch and a specific odour and sometimes consisting of only a few vesicles. This psora is the true underlying cause and the creator of almost all the multitudinous, indeed innumerable disease forms that are not due to syphilis and gonorrhea. They include neurasthenia, hysteria, hypochondria, mania, melancholia, idiocy, madness, epilepsy and all kinds of fits, softening of the bones (rachitis), scrofula, scoliosis and kyphosis, suppuration of the lungs, impotence and infertility, migraine, deafness, kidney stones etc. All these are mentioned in the pathology books as separate diseases. It took me twelve years of research to find the source of this incredible number of chronic diseases and to investigate and confirm this great hidden truth and to discover the principle anti-psoric remedies that are usually able to deal with this miasm in its widely varying forms and manifestations.

The anti-psoric remedies were presented by Hahnemann in Volume 2 of *The Chronic*

Diseases and included such great **polycrests** as Sulphur, Pulsatilla, Rhus toxicodendron, Calcarea carbonica. The word 'polycrest' (or polychrest) was coined by Hahnemann from the Greek words 'poly' (many) and 'crestos' (uses). Thus, the polycrests are defined as remedies with many uses, that is they may be used to treat a wide range of common symptoms and they are widely used in homoeopathy. It is important to realize that they are polycrests because they induced many common symptoms in their original 'provings' on healthy people.

Commenting on Hahnemann's teaching, Dr Roberts stated 'the very ear marks of the various stigmata show their respective characters. The psoric itches appear to be unclean and unwashed. The syphilitic ulcerates and the body structure is changed. The psychotic infiltrates and is corroded and by its discharges.'

Like Hahnemann he believed that all three miasms were destructive over mind, body and spirit. In Hahnemann's time it was claimed that while 10 per cent of the population contracted syphilis and 8 per cent contracted gonorrhea, no less than 82 per cent suffered from psoric diseases. Hahnemann's great biographer, Dr Richard Haehl, said that, to Hahnemann, 'the psora is a disease or disposition to disease hereditary from generation to generation for thousands of years and it is the fostering soil for every possible disease condition'. In his book *The Chronic Miams*, psora and pseudo psora, G.H. Allen wrote that 'for thousands of years the psora has disfigured and tortured mankind'.

Today miasmic theory would be studied in terms of the genetic code and dioxyribonucleic (DNA) and ribonucleic (RNA) acid structures, that determine hereditary characteristics.

New Miasms

During the twentieth century two new miasms have been identified, namely the **tubercular** and **carcinosin** miasms. It is now also recognized that miasms can be acquired rather than inherited, for example in blood transfusions or through the abuse and over-use of modern drugs, including antibiotics, contraceptives, fertility drugs and vaccination.

Anti-Miasmic Treatment

Thus, these chronic diseases lie dormant in the body – are susceptible – and can be

Miasm	Principle Remedy	Nosode
Sycotic (gonorrhea)	Thuja occidentalis	Medorrhinum
		(Leuticum)
Syphilitic (syphilis)	Mercurius solubulis	Syphilinum
Psoric (the itch)	Sulphur	Psorinum
Tubercular (tuberculosis)		Tuberculinum
Carcinosin (cancer)		Carcinosin

activated according to our sensitivity. Miasms may be treated homoeopathically with high or very high potencies to penetrate deep enough to act upon the genetic code. It has been reported that such treatments should commence and finish with the remedy Sulphur, and doses are best given in the morning on rising.

Anti-Psoric Remedies

The main classical anti-psoric remedies associated with the nosode **Psorinum** (see chapter 8) are: Alumina, Arsen alb., Baryta carb., Calc phos., Crotalus, Graphites, Kali. carb., Lac. can., Nat. sulph. Pyrogen, Apis mel., Arsen. iod., Bufo, Carbo an., Hepar sulph., Kali. Iod., Lachesis, Natrum ars., Acid nit., Aurum net., Calc. carb., Carbo veg., Lodum, Ledum, Nat. carb., Secale, Anarcardium, Aurum mur., Cal. an., Capsicum, Conium, Acod fleur, Kali. bich., Lycopodium, Nat. mur., Phosphorus, Selenium, Sepia, Sulphur, Silicea, Staphisagria, Tarantula and Zincum Met.

Anti-Sycotic (Gonorrhea) Remedies

Associated with the nosode **Medorrhinum** (see chapter 8) are: Ledum, Lycopodium, Mezereum, Nat. mur., Sepia, Kali. bich., Nat. sulph., Silicea, Ars. alb., Calc. ars., Kali. carb., Nat. ars., Acid nit., Progen, Staphisagria, Ars. iod., Causticum, Kali. iod., Nat Carb., Phosphorus, Thuja (see Chapter 5).

Anti-Syphilic Remedies

Associated with the nosode **Syphilinum** are: Calc. ars., Kali. carb., Merc. sol., Staphysagria, Kali. iod., Acid nit., Aurum met., Hepar sulph., Lachesis, Aurum mur., Lycopodium.

Tubercular Remedies

Associated with the nosode **Tuberculinum** (see chapter 8) (Tub Bov, Tub Aviare, Tub Pisces) are: Phosphorus, Nux vom., Calc. phos., Calc. Carb. (see Chapter 8).

CONSTITUTION

Although it barely featured in Hahnemann's *Organon of Medicine* the concept of constitutional prescribing had been mooted by Hahnemann's predecessor, Paracelsus (1493–1531), 'All man's diseases originate in his constitution. It is necessary to know his constitution if we wish to know his disease.'

Hahnemann did refer obliquely to this concept, in the Organon, paragraph 5: 'The homoeopathic practitioner should consider the physical constitution of the patient, his affective and intellectual character, his activities, his way of life, his habits, his family relationships, his age, his sexual life.'

In paragraphs 211 to 213 of the *Organon*, Hahnemann commented: 'The mental and emotional constitution of a patient may be a decisive factor in the choice of the remedy'.

In Hahnemann's other works he made such comments as, 'Aconite will seldom, or never, cure if the disposition of the patient is calm and undisturbed'. He also wrote, 'Nux vomica will not cure the mild and phlegmatic patient'; 'Pulsatilla will not cure the cheerful or wilful'; 'Ignatia will not cure if the patient is steady without fear or irritability.'

Hahnemann also wrote of the 'indescribable diversity and distinct congenital constitution'. These references linking remedies to the disposition or the personality of the patient may be seen as the forerunner to the concept of constitution.

However, we owe the development of the concept of constitution to Dr James Tyler

Kent in America, and Dr Margaret Tyler and Dr Margery Blackie in the UK in early part of the twentieth century. It was not introduced by one specific paper, but rather evolved through the publication of a series of 'drug pictures' over several years, which laid increasing emphasis on the physical, emotional and psychological features of the patient rather than the pathological symptoms.

In his Lesser Writings, Kent wrote: 'To the homoeopathic practitioner: Ten years of practice will be a revelation to you so that you will understand people and their minds. You will almost know what they are thinking and often take in a patient's **constitution** at first glance.'

Dr William Osler encapsulated the constitutional approach when he instructed his students, 'Ask yourself not what kind of disease the patient has, but what kind of patient has the disease'.

Dr Margery Blackie, who, before the doctor's death, had been physician to HM Queen Elizabeth II, once told the author that she could often decide on a patient's constitution in the first five minutes, even by a handshake. In practice, determining a patient's 'constitutional type' is usually much more difficult, but in Dr Kent's and Dr Blackies' case this was probably a fair comment.

Concept of Constitution

In the first two decades of the twentieth century physicians gradually gave constitutional factors more and more consideration. The concept of constitution, therefore, is that certain types of people have a special affinity for a particular medicine (or vice versa) and will respond positively to it.

In determining the patient's constitution the physician is concerned not only with his or her physical characteristics, such as colour of hair, colour of eyes, physique, deportment, but also the mental, emotional and psychological characteristics such as sensitivity, intelligence, restlessness or moods.

This approach seemed anathema to many classical homoeopaths who based their practice of homoeopathy on Hahnemann's teaching of the Law of Similars. Kent, however, believed that individuals respond best to the Similimum within a constitutional model.

It led inevitably to a bitter conflict with those physicians who followed the teachings of Hahnemann and the strict application of the Similimum based on pathological symptoms. The schism became even wider when Kent's teaching called for the administration of very high potencies (see Chapter 3) in constitutional prescribing. As we have seen in Chapter 1, this led to Dr Richard Hughes in the UK, an adherent to the use of low potencies, to describe Kent's potencies as being so high as to be 'airy nothings'. Kent retorted that Hughes's potencies were so low that they were 'practically allopathic'. This public conflict was seized upon by the detractors of homoeopathy and certainly contributed to its decline in the first half of the century.

To sum up this point:

1 Constitutional factors may lead to the choice of a different remedy for different people suffering from the same diseases.
2 The constitutional remedy may be the same as the remedy chosen to the Similimum. This might be considered to be the ideal situation as it satisfies both the pathological and the constitutional approach to prescribing.
3 It may seem to be stating the obvious, but

constitutional features are not symptoms. Thus, for example, it is not possible to make a mean person generous nor a poor-time keeper punctual.

4 The constitution or 'make up' of a person is fixed in their genes at birth and it cannot be changed except peripherally through the exigencies of life, for example, child abuse, environmental factors, traumatic experiences etc.

Constitution of the Remedy, Lachesis

As an example of a constitution, let us consider that of the polycrest remedy, Lachesis mutus. This remedy has what is described as a strong constitution and it illustrates many striking features. *The keynote is over stimulation.*

Potential energy not being released is the prime cause of a Lachesis person's problems. Anything that prevents the Lachesis person expending his or her pent-up energy and emotion causes problems, for example suppressed sexual desire.

Physically the Lachesis type is a dark, spare, over-active person with a pale complexion, bulbous and dull red nose. They may be a redhead with freckles. The face may acquire a purplish or bloated, congested look and will be hot to the touch. The Lachesis person has a distinctly suspicious, even furtive look, with thin, unsmiling lips and glazed, unblinking eyes. The tongue may be slimy and tremulous. Lachesis people are prone to purplish, multi-coloured discolorations or mottling of the skin with foul-smelling discharges. They suffer very constrictive spasms, with much clutching of the throat.

Mentally they may be anxious and self-conscious. The eyes are wide open as if from fear. They are highly loquacious, darting from subject to subject without pause, with a lashing tongue such that they do not realize the hurt they give others. Their ever-active tongue, pouring forth a spate of words, is often slanderous. The Lachesis type tends to finish others' sentences. They will interrupt and go back to exactly where they were when they last spoke – 'Enough about me, now tell me about my latest book' typifies their egotistical manner. They also have an urge to confess to misdemeanours that they have never committed, simply to seek attention.

They are so egocentric that they are unable to laugh with those who laugh and unable to cry with those who cry. They may shed tears, not in sympathy, but for self-pity.

They are prone to alternating moods with unbearable anxiety, particularly on waking, when they are depressed, confused and disorientated, restless, hyper-sensitive, with suppressed emotion and sexuality which makes them unstable and unattractive. They are full of schemes, but rarely see things through to completion. They are suspicious, put the worst interpretation on innocent facts and always take a pessimistic view.

They are suspicious without cause, and the Lachesis patient's innate suspicion may cause them to refuse to take the remedy until he or she knows its source.

They are constantly finding fault with everything and everyone.

The Lachesis person has a very jealous nature. They are only interested in what you can do for them. They tend to 'suck people dry'. Their pre-meditated jealousy extends to getting other people into trouble deliberately when envy overwhelms them. This jealousy exacerbates their quarrelsome nature.

They are charismatic people who appreciate the finer things in life, but they are self-centred and selfish with a desire to be amused. They are extrovert and outgoing but at the same time can be dishonest and sneaky.

Lachesis people must do everything quickly, exemplified by a tendency to eat fast and gulp their food, with the result that they may suffer from belching and flatulence. They may have an insatiable thirst, especially for hot drinks.

Lachesis girls at puberty are inclined to be depressed, and can experience menstrual problems and difficult pregnancies.

All Lachesis people are conscious of any constriction about their neck or waist. They are liable to constantly tear at their collar to relieve this perceived restriction. All symptoms are better for swallowing, particularly with a desire to swallow solids rather than liquids.

There is tendency for symptoms to spread from left to right, and there is a strong left-sided laterality.

They may sweat profusely and all senses are intensified, particularly touch and noise.

They have a fear of going to sleep, a fear of lying down, and they sleep into aggravation. Their sleep is disturbed, possibly with nightmares and they can experience a sensation of their bed swaying from side to side. They may have cold hands and feet.

They may have a strange fear of 'something lurking behind them' and it is this fear that causes them to seek the back seat of a bus or a car.

The Lachesis type is always better in the evening and at night, and they may suffer from intense photophobia.

It may be significant that many Lachesis features resemble those of the snake from whose venom it is derived (see Chapter 7, Doctrine of Signatures).

Further details of the Lachesis constitution and the constitutions of other remedies are given in Chapter 8.

HIGH POTENCIES – AVOGADRO'S HYPOTHESIS

There is no greater criticism of homoeopathic medicine by allopathic physicians than that concerning the ramifications of Avogadro's hypothesis. This phenomenon is so fundamentally important in homoeopathic practice that it deserves the proper discussion that many textbooks avoid. The Italian physicist, Avogadro, postulated, in 1811, that equal volumes of substances contain equal numbers of molecules. Therefore, unit volume of $1cm^3$ (or 1ml) contains a specific number of molecules and this number he calculated as 6.4×10^{23} molecules (at standard temperature and pressure).

Since Avogadro's hypothesis was proved valid and is now part of scientific law, it must be conceded that the serial dilution used in the preparation of homoeopathic potencies has to ultimately 'dilute out' every molecule contained in the original volume of mother tincture.

Thus, by Avogadro's hypothesis, the original volume (1 ml) of mother tincture contains 6.4×10^{23} molecules.

Then, in the preparation of 1ml of the first decimal potency (1X) – a dilution of 1 in 10 – the number of molecules remaining is 6.4×10^{22} molecules. Continuing the decimal potentization procedure, this means:

1 ml of a 2X potency contains 6.4×10^{21} molecules of the original mother tincture,

1 ml of a 3X potency contains 6.4×10^{20} molecules and so on, until

1 ml of a 4X potency contains 6.4×10^{19} molecules of the original mother tincture, and so on until we reach

1 ml of a 23X potency contains 6.4 molecules (which, of course, is impossible).

Thus, 1 ml of a 24X potency contains no molecules of the original mother tinture.

Theoretically, therefore, a 24X potency with a dilution of the original mother tincture of 1×10^{24} cannot contain any molecules of the mother tincture. Obviously, all potencies higher than 24X, or 12C which have the same dilution (see Chapter 3), theoretically cannot contain any molecules of the mother tincture ingredients.

The detractors of homoeopathy see this as the Achilles' heel of homoeopathy. Believing that only massive macromolecular doses of the active substance (which may be highly toxic and induce iatrogenic disease) can cure, such detractors express their incredulity that dosing with no actual physical medicament can possibly have any therapeutic effect. They argue that in effect liquid homoeopathic potencies above 24X or 12C are simply a solution of alcohol and water. Not surprisingly homoeopathic research into this phenomenon has centred on establishing the proof that high potencies are more than solutions of alcohol and water, even though no 'active ingredient' remains.

The position may be summarized as follows:

1 Clinical data

There is massive clinical evidence of the successful treatment of millions of people with high potencies over nearly two hundred years. Many of these cases were not properly recorded but there is an on-going programme, initiated by the Faculty of Homoeopathy, of building up a database of statistical data, which demonstrates unequivacally the therapeutic effectiveness of high potencies.

2 Physical properties

This research has centred on measuring the physical properties of solutions of high potencies, such as viscosity, conductivity, optical activity and specific gravity, to establish differences when compared with properties of pure alcohol/water solutions. Little progress has been made with this approach, since even the most modern laboratory equipment is not accurate enough to detect the infinitesimally small differences involved.

3 Chemical properties

Considerable progress has been reported in investigations of the spatial arrangements of alcohol and water molecules (stereochemic configurations) in high potency solutions. The complex, three-dimensional structures of the atoms and molecules viewed spectroscopically indicate the existence of 'holes' of distinctive 'shapes' within the structure. These 'holes', which are not present in pure alcohol and water, suggest that their particular shape may be related to the original molecules of the mother tincture that have been 'diluted out' in potentizing . These may be regarded as the 'fingerprint' of the original molecules.

Further work by Barnard and Stevenson in the USA has produced evidence of molecular clusters forming specific patterns or 'electrochemical patterning' that may be related to the original mother tincture.

4 Spectroscopy

Early work studying the infra-red and ultra-violet spectra of high potency solutions failed to show any significant difference from pure alcohol water, probably due to lack of sensitivity. Callinan (1985), however, suggested that succussion (see Chapter 3) stores potential energy in the alcohol/water bonds that are in evidence in infra-red spectra. By far the most profound evidence of a distinction between high potency solutions and simple alcohol/water mixtures has been demonstrated with nuclear magnetic resonance (NMR) spectra. Young (1987) provided clear evidence that these resonance images showed that there was high-energy, sub-atomic activity in potencies above the Avogadro limit. Homoeopaths believe that these high potencies retain a link with the identify of the original mother tincture through a subtle energy that comes into play in the curative process.

AGGRAVATION

First it is important to differentiate between a *modality aggravation* and a *homoeopathic*

aggravation. The former relates to a worsening of the symptoms of a disease due to the influence of certain factors as perceived by a particular patient. The modality aggravation is therefore a highly individualized phenomenon (see Modalities below). The homoeopathic aggravation is a brief, slight worsening of the symptoms of the natural disease, which is related to the application of the Law of Similars. It is, therefore, of fundamental importance and it relates to every patient.

Hahnemann first hinted of homoeopathic aggravation when he discussed the Similimum in the *Organon*, paragraph 158, where he stated: 'If the remedy with the greatest number of matching symptoms to be covered in the disease being treated is used, then this

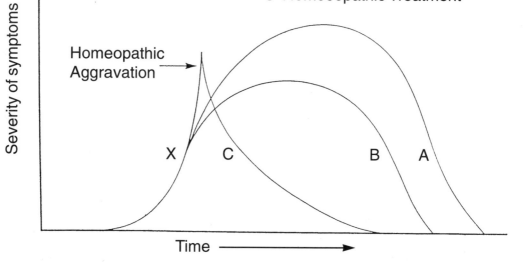

X Commencement of Treatment
A Untreated Disease
B Allopathic Treatment (suppression)
C Homoeopathic Treatment

Severity of symptoms

Homeopathic Aggravation

X   C   B   A

Time

Simplified Effect on Severity of Symptoms by Different Treatments remedy is the most suitable, and it will extinguish the disease with no ill effects.'

In paragraphs 156–158 of the *Organon* he was more specific:

Nevertheless, there is hardly any homoeopathic medicine, which during its action does not bring about some very slight unaccustomed complaint or small new symptom, particularly if the dose is too large. If the dose is too large, it is usual for the remedy to effect some small aggravation in the first hour or few hours after it is taken. This slight homoeopathic aggravation is a good portent.

Thus, Hahnemann admitted that on taking a homoeopathic medicine, however well chosen according to the Law of Similars, there is a strong likelihood that a slight worsening of the natural symptoms is almost inevitable. However, he suggests that this aggravation may indicate the correct choice of remedy with the closest matching proving symptoms. Putting it very simply this may be viewed as the induced similar symptoms of the artificial disease being superimposed momentarily over the symptoms of the natural disease before mutual elimination – the Law of Similars in action!

In practice there is only a slight worsening of the symptoms very briefly, possibly for only a fraction of a second and in nearly all cases it passes unnoticed by the patient. Thereafter the symptoms are reduced in their severity as healing proceeds. Thus, a slight, brief increase in the severity of symptoms may be seen as a precursor to cure. 'A good portent', as Hahnemann wrote.

Hahnemann squarely blamed a significant or noticeable aggravation on too high a dose (or too low a potency), as his prime concern was that a homoeopathic dose should not contain a significant material dose of a possibly toxic mother tincture or anything even approaching the massive macro doses of allopathy. He elaborated thus:

Because it is almost impossible for the [proving] symptoms of the chosen medicine and those of the [natural] disease to coincide exactly, there is hardly any homoeopathic remedy which does not bring about (especially in some sensitive patients) some very slight new symptom.

This facet of aggravation resulting in the

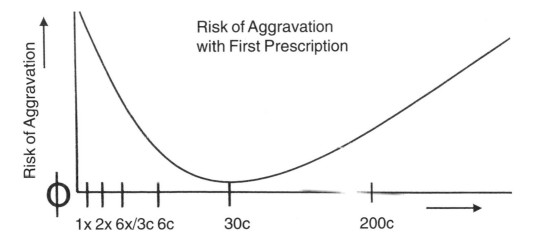

67

appearance of a new symptom suggests an unmatched, artificial, stronger symptom induced by the homoeopathic remedy. If the symptom persists then dosing must be stopped or a complementary remedy administered. The patient is said to be '*proving the remedy*'.

Kent advised: 'Do not prescribe the higher potencies [constitutionally] for hypersentive individuals or you may cause an aggravation.' Kent was aware of the risk at the other end of the potency scale with potencies of 1M or higher, where these penetrating, deep acting, high energy potencies can over-stimulate. Many an inexperienced practitioner who has boldly prescribed a potency of, say, 1OM or 5OM to a sensitive patient has learned a lesson when having to cope with a marked, prolongued aggravation.

The plussing technique (see Chapter X) offers a safer passage for the patient in terms of reduced risk of aggravation.

FREQUENCY OF DOSAGE

In *The Chronic Diseases* (1832), Hahnemann instructed that we should continue dosing with the same potency until the symptoms start to return or remain stationary and thus avoid a 'tumultuous aggravation'. Thus, each dose of every potency must be allowed to run its full therapeutic course, otherwise their action overlaps and the system may be over-stimulated.

In deciding the frequency of dosage, therefore, one should take into account the duration of action of the remedy. Thus, a fast-acting remedy with a short duration of therapeutic action may be given more frequently than a slow-acting remedy.

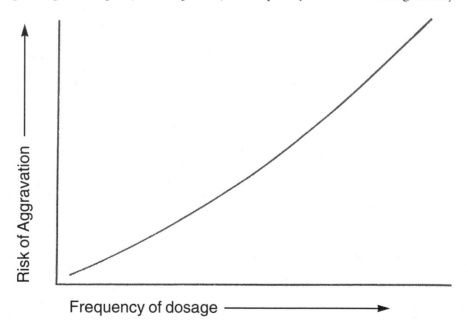

Relationship between Frequency of Dosage and Risk of Aggravation

Fast-acting remedies:

Aconite	1–2 hours' duration of action
Glonoine	1 day
Coffea	1–1½ days
Arum tryph	1–2 days

Thus, Aconite may be given in the appropriate potencies at a high frequency of dosage of, say, every hour for the first few hours with little risk of aggravation.

Slow-acting remedies:

Calc. phos.	60 days' duration of action
Graphites	40–50 days
Silicea	60 days
Thuja	60 days

Conversely these slow-acting remedies should be given at a low frequency of dosage to avoid overloading.

To summarize, the causes of aggravation can be found among the following:

1. Too high a dose (too low a potency).
2. Too high a potency.
3. Prescribing the wrong remedy, poorly matched by the Law of Similars.
4. Sensitive patients.
5. Correct remedy – the Law of Similars in action (a good portent!).
6. Too high a frequency of dosage.

Provings

Hahnemann took great care to ensure that the risks to the prover were minimal. For example, in a letter to his lifelong friend and fellow homoeopathic physician, Dr Stapf, he instructed:

I enclose some tincture of *Helleborus niger* which I gathered myself. Take one drop, in 8 ounces of water and a scruple of alcohol, shake it briskly and take one ounce before breakfast, continue thereafter as long as you are not too severely affected. Should severe symptoms occur, take some drops of tincture in camphor in one ounce of water.

In a tribute to these heroic experimenters, Dr Margaret Tyler wrote in 1931, 'For years, for half a lifetime, they had been proving drug after drug and suffering their effects in their minds and bodies'.

In spite of recent proving of new remedies, such as Lac Humanum (Melissa Assilem), Scorpion (Jeremy Sherr) and Musa Sapientum (Prakash Vakil), we still rely greatly on Hahnemann's remedies presented in his *Materia Medica Pura* (1811–1821) and *The Chronic Diseases*, Volume 2. With the infinite availability of natural substances, we should be carrying out more provings. Modern provings can benefit from the protocols of allopathic clinical trials by adapting the double-blind crossover technique with the use of a placebo. This is in no way incompatible with classical homoeopathic concepts. As Kent wrote: 'The best way to study a remedy is to make a proving of it'.

MODALITIES

In Hahnemann's *Organon* (at paragraph 133), he explained the manner in which the individual characteristics of a symptom were determined in the content of a homoeopathic proving:

In order to define a particular medicinal symptom with precision, it is helpful, indeed necessary to place oneself in varying circumstances and to observe whether the symptom increases, decreases or disappears from movement of the affected part, from walking indoors or in the open, from standing, sitting or lying, whether or not it tends to return when one reverts to earlier circumstances; whether it is modified by eating, drinking, speaking, coughing, sneezing or other bodily activities; at what time of the day or night it tends to be particularly evident. These modifying influences may be considered to be also appropriate when applied to the symptoms of the natural disease, as perceived by the patient and thereby direct us to the Similimum through the individual characteristics of the remedy.

A modality may be defined as a mode or influence that involves affirmation of possibity, but a simpler definition is that it is a factor which makes a symptom of a disease better or worse as perceived by the patient. In the context of homoeopathic treatment, since these modifying influences relate to each individual patient, its holistic approach is enhanced.

Worsening of a symptom is defined as an aggravation and is denoted by the symbol <.

Improvement of a symptom is defined as an amelioration and is denoted by the symbol >.

The modality aggravation must not be confused with the homoeopathic aggravation. The former relates to each individual patient, while the latter is of fundamental importance and relates to every patient, since it is governed by the Law of Similars (see Aggravation above).

Modalities are an essential tool in adequate case taking. Hahnemann described modalities as 'these singular and characteristic signs', and stressed their importance as an invaluable guide to the choice of a remedy.

Thus, if two or more remedies are equally indicated following the repertorization of the presenting symptoms, then modalities, whether aggravations or ameliorations, specific to one of these remedies as given in the Materia Medica are a strong pointer to its final choice. For example, if the choice lies between Petroleum, Sepia and Sulphur for a skin condition, then a modality 'worse in winter' would favour prescribing Petroleum.

Modalities may be associated with the causation of the symptoms or their effect on a particular part of the body, the mind, time or environmental factors. They may be classified as follows:

PHYSICAL: Symptoms are better or worse for touch, rest, motion, lying down, stooping, standing, walking, drawing up a limb, ascending or descending (stairs), sitting, on rising, on bending head.

TEMPERATURE: Symptoms are better or worse for hot, cold, warmth, cold air, drafts, warm applications, exposure.

TIME: Symptoms are better or worse during morning, afternoon, evening, night, hour of day or night, alternate days, periodic.

CLIMATE: Symptoms are better or worse for wet, damp, dry, cold winds, before or after thunderstorms, spring, summer, autumn, winter, by the seaside.

DIETARY: Symptoms are worse or better for eating, drinking (hot drinks or cold drinks), before or after eating, alcohol, coffee, fatty foods, spicy foods, fast foods, butter, pork, sweets, etc.

LATERALITIES (LOCALIZED): Symptoms are better or worse on right side, left side, right side moving to left side, left side moving to right side, radiating in certain directions.

MISCELLANEOUS: These modalities are unclassifiable. Examples are worse for music (Graphites, Thuja), worse for smoking (Aconite), worse after sleep (Apis mel.), worse for sweets or candies (Argent. nit.), worse for smoking (Ignatia, Staphysagria).

CLASSICAL HOMOEOPATHY

Hahnemann's concept of classical homoeopathy was set strictly within the bounds of the Law of Similars, prescribing the Similimum remedy as laid down in his Organon of Medicine (see Chapter 2).His instruction was quite clear: **'In no case being treated is it necessary to give a patient more than a single, simple medicinal substance at one time'** (Organon, paragraph 273). He was not against the use of other follow-up remedies in the course of the treatment if necessary, but only after each remedy had run its therapeutic course. He stressed the need for patience in the treatment.

K.D. Kanodia observed that Hahnemann clearly instructed that a dose of a single remedy be given on the basis of the totality of symptoms in the appropriate potency without undue repetition.

Hahnemann instructed that the appropriate potency should not be too low, that is not a significant material dose. Higher potencies are preferred (see Chapter 5).

Clearly the classical approach finds the use of combinations of two or more remedies given at the same time wholly unacceptable (see Chapter 9).

Summary of Classical Homoeopathy

To clarify the definition of classical Hahnemannian homoeopathy the main features may be summarized as follows:

1. A single remedy chosen according to the Law of Similars (the Similimum) is prescribed.
2. The *Organon of Medicine* is the infallible guide to homoeopathic treatment.
3. The appropriate homoeopathic remedy is chosen only in relation to the totality of the care.
4. Do not prescribe material doses.
5. Do not prescribe combination remedies.
6. Do not prescribe alternating remedies.
7. Do not use local applications, for example creams or suppositories.
8. Prescribe nosodes only where indicated.
9. Follow the concept of miasms.
10. Never use astrology, pendulums or electronic techniques in seeking the correct homoeopathic remedy.
11. Prescribe a single dose in high potency.
12. Wait after giving a prescription and then take the case again.

SUPPRESSION

Samuel Hahnemann often expressed his opposition to the suppressive nature of allopathic medicine. Suppression is defined as stifling, restraining, smothering, muffling, keeping back and checking normal development of symptoms. Suppression is not cure.

In the healthy state, the vital force is balanced and maintains a state of equilibrium in the body. External influences may, however, suppress the normal functioning of the vital force. Shock, fear or grief triggers a sequence of symptoms, which, if suppressed, will express themselves in a different pattern or return in a more severe form or even extend their effect into future generations. Medicines given in large doses result first in palliation then suppression as they prevent the natural expression of the disease.

An example is the suppression of a skin disease by topical applications of steroidal cream. The suppression camouflages the condition, in that is it has a cosmetic effect, but it does not cure. It may affect a chronic miasm which may be forced deeper to a vital organ. Thus, the sycotic miasm may lead to muscular and mucous problems by the use of sulphur ointment, while the syphilitic miasm may lead to metabolic disorders.

PALLIATION

Rather than restraining symptoms through suppression, palliation attempts the temporary removal of symptoms without achieving a cure. The administration of tranquilizers palliates the patient's symptoms but in doing so it reduces the power of the vital force. The result is the loss of the true picture of the disease and the demand for an increase in dosage.

Consider the palliation of pain. Pain is but part of the symptom picture and the homoeopathic practitioner must consider the exact location, the nature of the pain, its severity and its modalities.

Thus the path to cure is hampered by palliation. A homoeopathic remedy not selected on the basis of the Law of Similars has a palliating effect even if the condition is incurable.

SEQUENTIAL THERAPY

Rudolf Verspoor (*Homoeopathy Renewed*, 1998) stressed that to cure by the well-indicated homoeopathic remedy, the Similimum, is not in question. He believes, however, that after practising for some time the physician must face the reality that most chronic cases do not respond to the single, well-chosen remedy nor even a series of similar remedies. Following Hahnemann's example of a ceaseless quest for a cure, every means is employed, thereby sometimes deviating from the strict basic tenets of homoeopathy.

The concept of sequential therapy was introduced by the Swiss homoeopath, Dr Jean Elmiger. It is an extension of traditional homoeopathic practice, bringing together all the many facets of time in a patient's care history. In effect it introduces a new dimension into homoeopathic practice and is, therefore, contentious but at least worthy of open-minded discussion.

Rudolf Verspoor suggests that the constitutional or acute remedies are unable to overcome the major blockages underlying complex cases even if the symptom picture is approached on a 'layers' perspective or that of the essence or central disturbance. In sequential therapy, blockages need to be addressed from an etiological perspective, while keeping in mind the concept of illness through time in the correct sequence of events.

It can be argued that sequential therapy is not a new concept and does not deviate from the classical model: it simply draws attention to the importance of **time** which has an intrinsic role in homoeopathic practice.

Elmiger believed that unless major shocks were systematically examined, the vital force could not respond adequately to the well-indicated remedy in chronic cases. He set out these events or shocks in chronological order: birth traumas, natural childhood illness, vaccinations, traumatic life events, prolonged use of (allopathic) drugs and serious diseases (for example typhoid, cholera, malaria). These traumas are best treated in sequence.

In consideration of the role of time, Hahnemann's theory of chronic diseases and the inherited miasms naturally plays a part. Elmiger came to the conclusion that the classical nosodes, Psorinum, Tuberculinum, Medorrhinum and Luesinum, given in high potencies can act on the genetic code and sequential therapy is claimed to act in almost all chronic cases.

THE HIPPOCRATIC OATH

Historically the Hippocratic Oath, dating from 400BC, is the classical model of an ethical code of practice. In some ways it reflected the indentured apprentice system of training physicians. While the ideals of the Hippocratic Oath are as relevant today as they were in ancient times, the invocations and language are no longer appropriate.

After the Second World War the World Medical Association, formed in 1947 largely at the behest of the British Medical Association, adopted the Declaration of Geneva as being more appropriate in style to modern times. However, the ethos of the Hippo-cratic Oath is retained almost in its entirety. The Declaration of Geneva is thus a restatement of an international code of medical ethics which applies both in times of peace and war.

Surprisingly, while homoeopathy embraces the ideals of the Hippocratic Oath, homoeopaths have never formally adopted it.

In 1998 the affirmation of the Declaration of Geneva by new graduates of the British Institute of Homoeopathy in Homoeopathic Medicine became a public statement of their intent to maintain their high standards of ethical conduct and respect of learning.

At the time of becoming a practising trained homoeopath the Hippocratic Oath is as follows:

I solemnly pledge myself to consecrate my life to the service of humanity;

I will give to my teachers the respect and gratitude which is their due;

I will practise homoeopathy with conscience and dignity;

The health of my patient will be my first consideration;

I will respect the secrets which are confided in me, even after the patient has died;

I will maintain by all means in my power the honour and the noble traditions of homoeopathic medicine;

My colleagues will be my brothers and sisters; I will not permit consideration of religion, nationality, race, politics or social standing to intervene between my duty and patients;

I will maintain the utmost respect for human life from its beginning even under threat and I will not use my medical knowledge contrary to the laws of humanity;

I make these promises solemnly, freely and upon my honour.

DIFFERENTIAL DIAGNOSIS

Differential diagnosis helps bridge the gap between allopathic and homoeopathic medicine. Many practitioners are not taught diagnostic skills and the importance of distinguishing the severity of symptoms presented to them and many conditions do not fall into a clear-cut pattern, thus making it more difficult to distinguish more serious conditions. Differential diagnosis aims to give confidence in managing problematic symptoms and provide a deeper under-standing of severity and the need for referral.

Differential diagnosis is founded on a sound knowledge of anatomy and covers injuries, swellings, local infections, skin conditions, eye and face conditions, ear, nose and throat (ENT) and teeth problems, neck and back, extremities, chest conditions, abdomen, female problems, pregnancy, children's conditions, psychiatric conditions, occupational disease, endocrine system, rheumatic conditions and cancer.

CHAPTER 5

Case Taking

*Taking the case. Hering's Laws of Cure.
Hierarchy of symptoms. Repertorization.
Depth of symptoms. Prescribing. Choice of
potency. Case management. Concomitant
treatment. Role of the Practitioner.*

TAKING THE CASE

The essentials of homoeopathic case taking
were set out by Hahnemann in *The Organon
of Medicine* at paragraphs 83–104. He
stressed the importance of individualizing the
examination of a case of disease.

1. The patient tells the history of his or her
complaints (includes family history of
complaints).
2. The physician hears, sees and observes
with his or her other senses what is altered
and peculiar in the patient.
3. Write down everything exactly, including
verbatim expressions of the patient.
4. Remain silent – listen – let the patient
finish what he or she is saying, as long as
they do not digress unduly.
5. All symptoms should be written on
separate lines, one above the other on the
left-hand side of the paper, so that they
may be added to.
6. When the patient has finished speaking,
read through the list of symptoms and ask

for particulars. 'When did the symptom
appear?' 'Where was the pain exactly?'
'Was it continuous?' 'At what time of
day/night was it worse?'
7. Never put words into the patient's mouth.
For example, 'Was this circumstance also
present?' (paragraph 87).
8. Never ask a question that can be answered
'Yes' or 'No'. This encourages the patient
to affirm or otherwise out of a desire to
please. (It also provides the practitioner
with the least possible information.)
9. If information volunteered by the patient
omits mention of certain parts of the
body, the physician must ask if there is
anything to be said. For example, 'What
about your bowel movements?' 'What
about sleep?'.
10. More precise questions can then be
asked. For example: 'How frequent are
your bowel movements?'
11. When these statements are written
down, the physician records what he
himself observes in the patient. For
example, was the patient stressed?
Hoarse? Was there a rash? How dry was
the skin to touch?
12. Symptoms of a patient just after previous
allopathic treatment may not give a true
picture. (Hahnemann was well aware of
iatrogenic symptoms.) If the disease is
chronic, it could be left alone for a few

days (perhaps a placebo could be given).

13. If the disease is acute and so urgent as not to permit a delay, the physician must put together a symptom picture of the disease, regardless of alteration by other treatments.

14. Try to uncover any event that may have triggered a disease, for example alcohol, drugs, venereal disease or grief.

15. In cases of chronic disease, examine patient's day-to-day activities, for example diet or home circumstances or work.

16. In chronic diseases, investigation of symptoms must be thorough. When a patient has suffered for many years, they may have forgotten what health is or how it really feels!

17. Remember that different patients have different constitutional features and make allowances.

18. Questioning by the physician requires a high degree of tact, consideration, empathy, care and patience (paragraph 98).

19. Acute diseases are easier cases to take as they have arisen recently and the patient's memory is fresh and all symptoms are new.

20. Never assume a treatment in advance.

21. It is necessary to know the totality of symptoms to see the entire scope of the disease and grasp the homoeopathic remedy.

22. When the totality of symptoms is precisely written down, then the most difficult task is completed and the physician can find the Similimum.

HERING'S LAWS OF CURE

Constantine Hering, lifelong friend of Hahnemann, prover of Lachesis, Spigelia, Theridion and other remedies, and author of the ten-volume *Guiding Symptoms of the Materia Medica*, gave us three principles that are invaluable in evaluating the patient's state of health and monitoring their progress during treatment.

The three principles, sometimes known as the Laws of Direction of Cure, are

Depth of Symptoms

Mental	Emotional	Physical
Total confusion	Suicidal depression	Brain
Destructive delirium	Apathy	Heart
Delirium	Sadness	Endocrine glands
Paranoia	Anguish Liver	Delusions
Phobias	Lungs Lethargy	Anxiety
Kidneys	Dullness	Irritability
Bones	Lack of concentration	Dissatisfaction
Muscle	Forgetfulness	Skin
Absentmindedness		

as follows:

1. Healing proceeds from the deepest parts of the body – the mental and emotional levels and the organs – to the external parts, such as the skin and extremities.
2. As healing progresses, symptoms are cured in the reverse order of appearance.
3. Healing progresses from the upper parts of the body to the lower parts.

It follows that healing may be more apparent in deep-seated chronic conditions than in a superficial acute conditions.

Depth of Symptoms

In 1980 Vithoulkas produced a table listing the different depths or intensity of symptoms and their effects on health in descending order from the innermost to outmost. It serves as a useful guide in concert with Hering's Laws of Cure (see table).

REPERTORIZATION

From the publication of the first volume of Hahnemann's *Materia Medica Pura*, homoeopathic physicians called for a Repertory. Without a Repertory the practitioner must painstakingly proceed through the homoeopathic *Materia Medica*, remedy by remedy, from A to Z in order to obtain the best possible match of their proving symptoms with the similar presenting symptoms of the patient. Quite simply, a Repertory lists symptoms in alphabetical order and for each of these symptoms it presents a 'rubric' of remedies that induced the particular symptom in their proving.

Several Repertories, notably that by Bönninghausen, were produced in the nineteenth century and were limited to those homoeopathic remedies (mainly by Hahnemann) proved at that time. The first comprehensive Repertory, published in the early twentieth century, was the result of a monumental effort by James Tyler Kent and this is still used by the majority of homoeopathic practitioners today.

Several other Repertories were published in the late twentieth century, culminating in the *Complete Repertory*, by Roger Van Zandvoort, published in 1998 which embraces most other Repertories.

Repertories are now an intrinsic part of homoeopathic practice. Indeed it is considered that it is impossible to practise homoeopathy properly without the aid of a Repertory (see computer repertorization, Chapter 10).

The Kent Repertory breaks down the symptoms into thirty-one sections representing parts of the body or general symptoms: mind, vertigo, head, eye, vision, ear, hearing, nose, face, mouth, teeth, throat, expectoration, chest, back, extremities, sleep, chill, fever, perspiration, skin, generalities. It is supplemented by tables of *Relationship of Remedies, The Sides of the Body, Drug Affinities* and a word Index.

Lex Rutten (1991) provided some interesting statistics on Kent's Repertory. It covers about 650 homoeopathic medicines. It contains more than 60,000 rubrics. The occurrence of medicines throughout the Repertory is variable, in that 43 per cent occur in less than 100 rubrics and 32 per cent occur in 100–1000 rubrics.

The most common remedy is *Sulphur* which occurs in no less than 8,800 rubrics. The other polycrests occur in 5,000–7,000 rubrics.

The polycrests occur in 400/450 'Mind' rubrics. Indeed, the predominance of

Sulphur in the Repertory with its enormous range of proving symptoms prompts homoeopaths to claim that, if you repertorize long enough, you are bound to end up with Sulphur as the Similimum remedy!

HIERARCHY OF SYMPTOMS

The ranking, grading or hierarchy of symptoms is an important feature in case taking and repertorization.

The highest grade are **mental or mind symptoms** and they will always rule out those of lesser grades. Mental symptoms, however, must be definite and well marked if they are to be regarded as the most important symptoms of the case.

Mind symptoms may be categorized as follows:

1. Mental symptoms related to diseases of the nervous system, embracing intellect, judgement, perception and behaviour.
2. Psychological symptoms related to emotions, affections, willpower and desires.

The next highest grade are **general symptoms**, which relate to the patient and his or her reactions as a whole. The patient will say 'I have...' or 'I am...', for example 'I am frightened'. In this case the whole body is greater than the part.

The next highest grade are **particular symptoms**. These symptoms relate to any part of the body. The patient will say 'My leg hurts' or 'My fingers are numb'.

Particular symptoms are of the highest grade if they include anything strange, rare or peculiar. These symptoms are important because they usually are peculiar to a specific remedy. They are especially useful in acute cases and will often provide the answer when repertorizing has given a short list of drugs equally indicated.

Common symptoms, which are often present in a wide range of common, acute conditions, should be eliminated as they are of little value in repertorizing: they will complicate the repertorization as they are common to a large number of drugs. For example, the patient says 'I am thirsty'. Unless there is a clearly identifiable reason for the thirst, it can be misleading.

Particular symptoms, although of lesser value than general symptoms as a rule, are of greater importance when qualified by, say, exact location, sensations, modalities and comcomitants: for example, headaches, dull aching, open air, rest and lying down, motion ascending.

It is worth remembering that features relating to ego are always general, mental symptoms because they reflect the individuality of the patient. A general symptom can be constructed from a group of particulars carrying the same characteristic, for example, burning pain in the head, chest and abdomen – all relieved by hot applications. In this case the burning pain affects the patient as a whole and thus becomes a physical general symptom.

If the patient says 'It's as if...', then this clearly indicates that he or she is about to describe a **sensation**. An example might be, 'It's as if there were cobwebs on my face'. This sensation is peculiar to the remedy Graphites and it is a clear pointer to this remedy. It may be prescribed in preference to a more highly graded remedy.

The standard denotations of remedies in each rubric or sub-rubric of the Repertory are either in bold type or capitals as first grade, strongly indicated remedies; in italics as a second grade remedy or in plain type for a weakly indicated remedy.

Points are allocated to each type of remedy as follows:

CAPITALS or **Bold type** remedies	3 points
Italics remedies	2 points
Plain type remedies	1 point

Kent recommends a remedy with a strong laterality (see table, Sides of Body) denoted **bold type***, should be awarded 4 points. The sum of points awarded on this basis for each symptom repertorized is the prescribed remedy.

Examples of Repertorizing

The basic method is the taking of all the presenting symptoms and seeking all the associated remedies in rubrics or sub-rubrics with gradings. The sum of these gradings with modalities will indicate the appropriate remedy. This may be achieved manually or by using one of the several excellent computer repertorizing programs (see Chapter 10).

Let us consider some simple examples using the Kent Repertory.

Example 1

Presenting symptom: *Numbness around the eyes.*
Repertorizing, we find:

EYE. Page 235
then EYE. NUMBNESS around eyes. Page 247
The chosen remedy is **Asafoetida**.

Example 2

Presenting symptom and modality: *Bitter taste in the mouth at night.*
Repertorizing, we find:

MOUTH. page 397
then MOUTH. TASTE. page 422
then MOUTH. TASTE, bitter. page 422
then MOUTH. TASTE, bitter at night. page 422
The chosen remedy is **Lycopodium**.
Second choice is Antim. tart.

Example 3

Presenting symptom: *Quivering left upper eyelid.*
Repertorizing, we find:

EYE. page 235
EYE. QUIVERING. page 264
EYE. QUIVERING, lids. page 264
EYE. QUIVERING, left upper lid. page 264
Rubric: **Arum - t**, Berb, *Croc*
The chosen remedy is Arum triphyllum (3 points)
Second choice is crocus sativus (2 points)
A suggested **Repertorization Chart** for up to 10 rubrics is shown on pages 79–84.

SELECTION OF POTENCY IN HOMOEOPATHIC PRESCRIBING

In considering the choice of potency, we are reminded of the prime potencies which account for over 90 per cent of all prescriptions, namely 6X, 6C, 30C, 200C and 1M.

Eizayaga (1992) was probably correct in stating that there are as many views on potencies as there are homoeopaths. Textbooks tend to lack clear advice on this issue or include so many asterisks or footnotes that the advice is at best confusing. Even some of our greatest homoeopaths

Repertorization Chart

Case: rubrics	1	2	3	4	5	6	7	8	9	10
abies-c										
acon										
act-s										
aesc										
agar										
all-c										
aloe										
alum										
ambr										
am-c										
am-m										
anac										
ant-c										
ant-t										
apis										
arg-m										
arg-n										
arn										
ars										
ars-i										
arum-t										
aur										
aur-m										
bacc										
bapt										
bar-c										
bar-m										
bell										
bellis										
ben-ac										
berb										
bism										
bov										
brom										
bry										
cact										
calad										
calc-c										
calc-f										
calc-p										
calc-s										
camph										
cann-i										
canth										
caps										
carbo-a										
carbo-v										
caul										
caust										
cham										
chel										
china										
chin-a										
chin-s										
cimic										

	1	2	3	4	5	6	7	8	9	10
cina										
clem										
cocc										
coff										
colch										
coloc										
con										
crot-h										
crot-t										
cupr										
cupr-ar										
dig										
dios										
dros										
dulc										
eup-per										
euphr										
ferr										
ferr-ar										
ferr-p										
fl-ac										
gels										
glon										
graph										
ham										
hell										
hep										
hydr										
hyos										
hyper										
ign										
iod										
ip										
iris										
kali-ar										
kali-bi										
kali-c										
kali-m										
kali-p										
kali-s										
kalm										
kreos										
lac-c										
lach										
lac-ac										
led										
lil-t										
lob										
lyc										
mag-c										
mag-m										
mag-p										
mag-s										
mang										
med										
merc										
merc-c										
merc-ir										
merc-if										
mez										
mill										
mur-ac										
naja										

	1	2	3	4	5	6	7	8	9
nat-c									
nat-m									
nat-p									
nat-s									
nit-ac									
nux-m									
nux-v									
op									
ox-ac									
petro									
ph-ac									
phos									
phyt									
pic-ac									
plat									
podo									
psorn									
puls									
pyrog									
ran-b									
rhodo									
rhus-t									
rumex									
ruta									
sabad									
sabin									
sang									
sec									
sel									
sep									
sil									
spig									
spong									
stann									
staph									
stram									
stront									
stroph									
sulph									
sul-ac									
syph									
tab									
tarent									
ter									
thuja									
tub									
urt-u									
verat-a									
verat-v									
zinc									

Total Forward	Symptoms in numerical order with their Repertory Page / Remedies	1	2	3	4	5	6	7	8	9	10	11	12	Total	Total Forward		1	2	3	4	5	6	7	8	9	10	11	12	Total
	Abies-c.															Ap g.													
	Abies-n.															Apoc.													
	Abrot															Aral.													
	Absin.															Aran.													
	Aca.															Argc.													
	Acet-ac															Arg-m													
	Acon.															Arg-mur.													
	Acon-c.															Arg-n.													
	Acon-f.															Arn.													
	Act-sp.															Ars.													
	AEsc.															Ars-h.													
	AEth.															Ars-i.													
	Agar-em.															Ars-m.													
	Agar-															Ars-s-f.													
	Agar-ph.															Ars-s-r.													
	Agn.															Art-v.													
	Ail.															Arum-d.													
	Alet.															Arum-m.													
	All-c.															Arum-t.													
	All-s.															Arund.													
	Aloe.															Asat.													
	Alumn.															Asar.													
	Alum															Asc-c.													
	Alum-m															Asc-t.													
	Ambr.															Asim.													
	Ammc.															Aspar													
	Amph.															Astac.													
	Am-br.															Aster.													
	Am-c.															Atro.													
	Am-caust.															Aur.													
	Am-m															Aur-m.													
	Amyg.															Aur-m-n.													
	Aml-n.															Aur-s.													
	Anac																												
	Anag.															Bad													
	Anan.															Bapt													
	Ang.															Bart.													
	Anis.															Bar-ac.													
	Anth.															Bar-c.													
	Anthr.															Bar-m													
	Ant-a															Bell.													
	Ant-c.															Bell-p.													
	Ant-ox.															Benz.													
	Ant-s.															Benz-ac.													
	Ant-t.															Benz-n.													
	Aphis.															Berb.													
	Apis.															Bism.													
		1	2	3	4	5	6	7	8	9	10	11	12				1	2	3	4	5	6	7	8	9	10	11	12	

Total Forward		1	2	3	4	5	6	7	8	9	10	11	12	Total	Total Forward		1	2	3	4	5	6	7	8	9	10	11	12	Total
	Blatta															Chin-s.													
	Bol.															Chion.													
	Bor.															Chlol.													
	Bor-ac.															Chlf.													
	Both.															Chlor.													
	Bov.															Chr-ac.													
	Brach.															Clc.													
	Brom.															Cimx.													
	Bruc.															Cimic.													
	Bry.															Cina.													
	Bufo.															Cinch.													
	Buf-s															Cinnb.													
																Cinnm.													
	Cact.															Cist.													
	Cadm.															Cit-ac.													
	Cahin.															Cit-i													
	Caj.															Cit-v.													
	Calad.															Clem													
	Calc-ac.															Cob.													
	Calc-ar.															Coca.													
	Calc.															Cocc.													
	Calc-caust.															Coc-c.													
	Calc-f.															Coch.													
	Calc-i.															Cod.													
	Calc-p.															Coff.													
	Calc-sil.															Coff-t.													
	Calc-s.															Colch.													
	Calo.															Coll.													
	Camph															Coloc.													
	Cann-i															Com.													
	Cann-s.															Con.													
	Canth.															Cond.													
	Caps.															Conv.													
	Carb-ac.															Cop.													
	Carb-an.															Cor-r													
	Carb-h.															Cori-f.													
	Carbo-o.															Corn.													
	Carb-s.															Corn-f.													
	Carb-v.															Corn-s.													
	Card-m															Corc.													
	Carl.															Cort-c.													
	Casc.															Cort h.													
	Cast-v.															Cort-t													
	Cast-eq.															Cub.													
	Cast.															Culx.													
	Caul.															Cupr.													
	Caust.															Cupr.ar.													
	Cean.															Cupr-s.													
	Cedr.															Cur.													
	Cench.															Cycl.													
	Cent.															Cypr.													
	Cer-b.																												
	Cer-s.															Daph.													
	Cham.															Der.													
	Chel.															Dig.													
	Chen-a.															Dios.													
	Chen-v.															Dirc.													
	Chim.															Dol.													
	Chin.															Dorl.													
	Chin-a															Dros.													
		1	2	3	4	5	6	7	8	9	10	11	12				1	2	3	4	5	6	7	8	9	10	11	12	

81

Total Forward		1	2	3	4	5	6	7	8	9	10	11	12	Total	Total Forward		1	2	3	4	5	6	7	8	9	10	11	12	Total
	Dulc.															Hydr.													
																Hydrang.													
	Echi.															Hydr-ac.													
	Elaps.															Hydrc.													
	Elat.															Hyosh.													
	Epig.															Hyper.													
	Equis.																												
	Erig.															Iber.													
	Ery-a.															Ign.													
	Eucal.															Ill.													
	Eug.															Ind.													
	Euon.															Indg.													
	Eup-per															Indul.													
	Eup-pur.															Iod.													
	Euph.															Iodof.													
	Euphr.															Ip.													
	Eupi.															Ipom.													
																Irfl.													
	Fago.															Ir-foe													
	Ferr-ar.															Iris.													
	Ferr.																												
	Ferr-i.															Jab													
	Ferr-ma.															Jac.													
	Ferr-m.															Jal.													
	Ferr-p.															Jtar.													
	Ferr-pic.															Jug-c.													
	Ferr-s.															Jug-r.													
	Fl-ac.															Juni.													
	Form.																												
																Kali-ar.													
	Gamb.															Kali-bi.													
	Gels.															Kali-br.													
	Genist.															Kali-c.													
	Gent-l.															Kali-hi													
	Gent-c.															Kali-cy.													
	Ger.															Kali-fer.													
	Gins.															Kali-i.													
	Glon.															Kali-ma.													
	Gnaph.															Kali-n.													
	Goss.															Kali-p.													
	Gran.															Kali-s.													
	Graph.															Kalm.													
	Grat.															Kaol.													
	Grin.															Kiss.													
	Guar.															Kreos.													
	Guare.																												
	Guaj.																												
	Gymn.																												
																Lac-c.													
																Lac-d.													
	Haem.															Lac-f.													
	Ham.															Lach.													
	Hecla.															Lachn.													
	Hell.															Lac-ac.													
	Helo.															Lact.													
	Helon.															Lam.													
	Hep.															Lap-a.													
	Hippoz.															Lath.													
	Hipp.															Lat-m.													
	Ho.															Laur.													
	Hura.															Lec.													
			1	2	3	4	5	6	7	8	9	10	11	12				1	2	3	4	5	6	7	8	9	10	11	12	

Total Forward	Remedy	1	2	3	4	5	6	7	8	9	10	11	12	Total	Total Forward	Remedy	1	2	3	4	5	6	7	8	9	10	11	12	Total
	Led.															Nit-ac.													
	Lem-m.															Nit-m-ac.													
	Lepi.															Nit-s-d.													
	Lept.															Nuph.													
	Lil-t.															Nux-m.													
	Lith.															Nux-v.													
	Lith-m.																												
	Lob-c.															Oci.													
	Lob.															Œna.													
	Lob-s															Olnd.													
	Lyc.															Ol-an.													
	Lycpr.															Ol-j.													
	Lycps.															Onos.													
	Lyss.															Op.													
																Orig.													
	Mag-c.															Osm.													
	Mag-m.															Ox-ac.													
	Mag-p.															Oxyt.													
	Mag-s.																												
	Mag-ars.															Paeon.													
	Mag-aust.															Pall.													
	Maland.															Pareir.													
	Manc.															Par.													
	Mang.															Pen.													
	Mang-m.															Petl.													
	Med.															Petr.													
	Meli.															Petros.													
	Meny.															Phal.													
	Meph.															Phase.													
	Merc.															Phel.													
	Merc-c.															Ph-ac.													
	Merc-cy.															Phos.													
	Merc-d.															Phys.													
	Merc-i-f.															Phyt.													
	Merc-i-r.															Pic-ac.													
	Merc-n.															Pin-s.													
	Merc-sul.															Pip-m.													
	Merl.															Pip-n.													
	Mez.															Plan.													
	Mill.															Plat.													
	Mit.															Plat-m.													
	Morpin.															Plect.													
	Mosch.															Plb.													
	Murx.															Plumbg.													
	Mur-ac.															Podo.													
	Mygal.															Polyg.													
	Myric.															Pop.													
	Myris.															Poth.													
																Prun.													
	Naja.															Psor.													
	Narcot.															Ptel.													
	Nat-ac.															Pulx.													
	Nat-a.															Puls.													
	Nat-c.															Pul-n.													
	Nat-h.															Pyrog.													
	Nat-m.															Pyrus.													
	Nat-n.																												
	Nat-p.															Rad.													
	Nat-s.															Ran-b.													
	Nicc.															Ran-s.													
		1	2	3	4	5	6	7	8	9	10	11	12				1	2	3	4	5	6	7	8	9	10	11	12	

83

Total Forward		1	2	3	4	5	6	7	8	9	10	11	12	Total	Total Forward		1	2	3	4	5	6	7	8	9	10	11	12	Total
	Raph.															Tarent.													
	Rat.															Tarent-c.													
	Rheum.															Tax.													
	Rhod.															Tell.													
	Rhus-a.															Tep.													
	Rhus-t.															Ter.													
	Rhus-r.															Teucr.													
	Rhus-v.															Thal.													
	Rob.															Thea.													
	Rumx.															Ther.													
	Ruta.															Thuj.													
																Til.													
	Sabad.															Trif-p.													
	Sabal.															Tril.													
	Sabin.															Trom.													
	Sal-ac.															Tub.													
	Sal-n.															Tus-f.													
	Samb.															Tus-p.													
	Sang.																												
	Sanic.															Upa.													
	Sarr.															Uran.													
	Sars.															Urt-u.													
	Scut.															Ust.													
	Sec.															Uva.													
	Sei.																												
	Senec.															Vac.													
	Seneg.															Valer.													
	Senn.															Vario.													
	Sep.															Verat.													
	Sil.															Verat-v.													
	Sin-a.															Verb.													
	Sin-n.															Vesp.													
	Sol-m.															Vib.													
	Sol-n.															Vinc.													
	Sol-o.															Viol-o.													
	Sol-t-ae.															Viol-t.													
	Spg.															Vip.													
	Spig-m.															Visc.													
	Spira.																												
	Spong.															Wye.													
	Squil.																												
	Stach.															Xan.													
	Stann.																												
	Staph.															Yuc.													
	Stel.																												
	Stict.															Zing.													
	Still.															Ziz.													
	Sram.															Zinc.													
	Stront.															Zinc-m.													
	Stry.															Zinc-s.													
	Sulph.																												
	Sul-i.																												
	Sul-ac.																												
	Sumb.																												
	Syph.																												
	Tab.																												
	Tanac.																												
	Tann.																												
	Tarax.																												
			1	2	3	4	5	6	7	8	9	10	11	12				1	2	3	4	5	6	7	8	9	10	11	12	

differed in their views. There are relatively few ground rules on the choice of the correct potency for an individual case and homoeopathic practitioners tend to build up their own personalized approach, based on sound experience.

Let us first consider some wise general guidance on the subject:

The question arises what is the ideal degree of smallness? How small should the dose of a given correctly chosen homoeopathic medicine be to cure in the best way?
Only pure experiment, the meticulous observation of the sensitivity of each patient and sound experience can determine this in each individual case.
Hahnemann, Organon

If I start high, I have nowhere to go.
Geoffrey Martin, former president of the Faculty of Homoeopathy

High potencies are like a shower of rain on all the garden, and low potencies are like the watering can in some corner [of the garden] to overcome a local problem.
Dr Margery Blackie

In acute fevers one can repeat the doses of the lowest potencies at short intervals.
Hahnemann, Organon, paragraph 270

The most similar remedy does not become the Similimum until the potency is adjusted to the plane of the individual during his or her illness at the time of prescribing.
Elizabeth Hubbard

A homoeopath should know the whole range of potencies and when to use them. There is an almost endless field here for speculation and observation ranging from tinctures to the highest potencies.
Kent, Philosophy

The guiding principle is the degree of clarity. If you cannot decide between two or more remedies due to lack of clarity, prescribe only a 30C or a 200C potency: A higher potency can be given if there is a greater degree of certainty.

Vithoulkas

I prefer to start with lower potencies and adopt the 'Plus Method'.

Eizayaga, Treatise

The last two quotations given above (from Vithoulkas and Eizayaga) refer specifically to the 'plus' or 'plussing' method or technique, which is now used extensively by homoeopathic practitioners. Based on decimal and centesimal potencies, it draws on the serial prescriptions from the lowest LM potency (LM1) to the highest (LM30) introduced by Hahnemann in the sixth edition of his Organon (see Aggravation in Chapter 4).

Kent's philosophy was that a chronic case would be relieved by moderately high potencies (30C or 200C), but would only improve for a matter of weeks. However, on the administration of much higher potencies, the work would be taken up and in that way the same patient could be carried from one potency to another. In effect he was suggesting a 'plussing' method even before the introduction of LM potencies in the sixth edition of the Organon published some twenty years later.

The table on the next page gives guidelines on the choice of potency and the frequency of dosage in homoeopathic prescriptions. It is subject to infinite variation in individualized treatment and should be viewed only

HOMOEOPATHIC PRESCRIBING CHOICE OF POTENCY

	Initial Potency	Frequency of dosage	Remarks
Allergens	30C	Daily-at onset	Example: Mixed grass pollen. Daily prophylactic
Bowel Nosodes	30C	One dose (repeated after 3 months if necessary)	Paterson suggested IM if mental symptoms predominate
Organotherapy	4C, 6C, (low)*	Daily	Stimulatory
	7C (medium)	Daily	Regulatory
	12C, 30C (high)	Daily	Depressant
Gemmontherapy	2X	4-5- doses/day	2X only
Lithotherapy	8X	Daily	8X only
Drainage	1X, 2X, 3X	Hourly/3 daily	φ in some cases
Biochemic Tissue Salts	3X, 6X	3X daily	Triturated tablets
Topical Application	0 or 1X	As required	Includes creams
Cyclical/Periodic Symptoms		30C	3X daily
Acute disease	6X, 6C, 30C	HIGH - Initially hourly then 3 - 4X daily	
Physical symptoms	6X, 6C	HIGH - Initially hourly then 3 - 4X daily	
Chronic Disease	200C, 1M	LOW - Every other day, twice a week	
Mental Symptoms	200C, 1M	LOW - Every other day	
Constitutional Prescribing	1M, 10M, 50M	VERY LOW - One dose. Repeat after 1 month, 3 months, or 6 months	
Very Painful Cases	Very Low 2X, 3X, 6X	Hourly	For example, Lithaisis
Infants	Low 6C, 30C	3X daily	Preferably Centesimal potencies
low Vitality Patients	Low 6X, 12X, 6C	Hourly or 4X daily	Elderly people
Very Sensitive Patients	Low or Medium 6C, 30C		3X daily 'Prove' every remedy given
Terminal Conditions	Low		

*(Definition corresponds to French practise)

as a grounding as there are no precise rules. Summarizing:

Wrong remedy + Wrong potency = No cure. Aggravation!
Wrong remedy + Right potency = No cure.
Right remedy + Wrong potency = Some improvement. Aggravation possible.
Right remedy + Right potency = Cure.
Thus, to put the choice of potency into perspective, important though it is, the choice of the correct Similimum remedy overrides any other consideration.

Potencies	
Low	3x, 6x, 12x, 6C, 24x
Medium	30x, 30C, 200x
High	200C, 1M
Very High	10M, 50M, CM

CONCOMITANT TREATMENT

Iatrogenic Disease

It is necessary to ascertain what allopathic drugs have been or are being taken by the patient, not only to face the decision whether to discontinue (a decision which must be taken with caution), but also to determine whether the patient is suffering from side-effects. Treatment of iatrogenic disease may be a precursor to homoeopathic treatment, as its symptoms inevitably confuse the symptom picture. Determining which of the presenting symptoms are a manifestation of the natural or the iatrogenic

disease may be difficult, but reference to the British National Formulary or its American equivalent is useful.

Importance of Lifestyle

When he practised in Paris, Hahnemann invariably gave his patients a diet sheet along with their homoeopathic medicine. He had advocated the need for a healthy lifestyle as early as 1795, when he wrote in his work, *The Friend of Health*:

Fresh air, fresh water, free movement are, as a general rule, always the preliminary condition of well being. Next to food, exercise is the most essential requirement of the human mechanism – it is that alone which winds up the machinery. Exercise and good air alone set all the humours in our body in motion to fill their appointed places and compel every secreting organ to give off its specific secretions to give power to the muscles and to the blood. They refine the fluids so they alone best invite us to rest and sleep which is the time of refreshment for the production of new spirit and energy.

Patients (or clients) of the homoeopathic practitioner must not be passive. They should be totally involved in their treatment and be prepared to change their habits or lifestyle in their determination by sheer willpower to regain their health. In this way the body's natural immune system is optimized and the homoeopathic remedy has the best chance of success. Conventional medicine has encouraged patients to demand 'instant cure' and by suppression of disease symptoms they are enabled to resume the lifestyle that was probably the cause of their condition in the first place.

Anything that is contrary to a person's harmony with nature can lower his or her immunity against disease. The health risks associated with stress, anxiety or fear over a prolonged period are well known. Pollution is another increasing problem, not only from airborne pollutants but also from toxic food additives, drugs and even dental fillings.

Role of the Practitioner

Empathy and compassion are synonymous with the homoeopathic approach: there is no place for the rude, intolerant, impatient, uncaring practitioner. If patients leave the consulting room knowing that the practitioner cares, the cure is already under way. The practitioner needs to develop the potential for caring, responsiveness and adaptability before he or she is able to help others. Mechanistic case taking, even if it involves a brilliant repertorizing technique and an expert knowledge of the Materia Medica is not enough.

The practitioner must be involved beyond the prescription by helping patients to improve the quality of their lives and remove those things which depress or stress them. For example, it would be wholly in keeping with the homoeopathic ethos to suggest that a long-term unemployed patient suffering from depression should prepare a curriculum vitae as the first step to a new resolve to find a job (and at the same time take the first step to their recovery).

The value of a sense of humour and particularly laughter should not be under-estimated. The body and mind are never more totally relaxed than when we are laughing.

Dr Pietroni (1984) encapsulated the role of the homoeopathic practitioner when he urged that we should replace the mechanistic approach to the study of health and disease with a humanistic approach, where sharing, caring, loving, touching and hoping play an important role in our endeavours.

THE DECLARATION OF GENEVA

Historically, the **Hippocratic Oath**, dating from 400BC, is the classical model of an ethical code of practice.In some ways it reflected the indentured apprentice system of training physicians.

While the ideals of the Hippocratic Oath are as relevant today as they were in ancient times, the invocations and language are no longer appropriate.

After the Second World War, the World Medical Association, formed in 1947 largely at the behest of the British Medical Association, adopted the Declaration of Geneva as being more appropriate in style to our times. However, the ethos of the Hippocratic Oath is retained almost in its entirety. The Declaration of Geneva is thus a restatement of an international code of medical ethics which applies both in times of

CHAPTER 6
Case Studies

Actual cases and their homoeopathic treatment.

This chapter presents a selection of actual case studies chosen to illustrate many facets of homoeopathy and the diversity of case-taking techniques adopted by individual practitioners. Some cases are provided by Dr Anita Pride, Bruce Berkowsky and Peter Quenter, to whom I am indebted.

CASE 1

Date: 16 August
Female
Age: 83, brought in by her daughter

Small physical build, white hair, many wrinkles in her face but looks rather like an energetic elderly lady if it were not for the tired posture she takes on the chair, she seemed friendly and gentle right from the start.

Present complaint is sinus trouble which has been going on all through summer. 'I'm fed up with this', are her words. Usually she has the problem treated repeatedly with antibiotics, and she does not know why the problem persists now also in summer. When she was younger she had hay fever, which improved when she lived for many years up in the north of the country. After moving to Ottawa her winter-sinus trouble began a common occurrence, it seems, in the Ottawa area. People moving here from different parts of the world experience onset of hay fever, asthma, catchcall symptoms.

Details are: pressure in the forehead, mucous build up with postnasal drip, lots of thick, yellow mucous. <heat, humidity, tea, coffee, chocolate pudding (which certainly is a common symptom), she stopped eating cheese already on her own, her energy is down and she has lost weight. She also has frequent belching daily, because of which she recently avoids going out of the house or talking to people, she says generally she does not talk about illness because she's never really been ill and she would rather be active and get things done, so all this is not at all her usual self and being house-bound only makes her worse.

She has a cataract in her right eye, three months ago she fell and fractured her left arm, she is nervous going to the doctor, takes medication for high blood pressure, a diuretic and a thyroid medication.

Prescription

Arnica 200 – 1M – 10M three consecutive evenings because of the recent physical trauma (fracture).

Additionally: Tissue salts Kali. mur. 6X, Kali. sulf. 6X, Nat. mur. 6X, these for the sinuses; Calc. phos. 6X for bone healing. All four approx. three tabs twice per day each, for about two months, on the fourth day (the day after Arnica 10M) starting Hydrastis 6X approx. 5 drops twice per day for drainage, one week after visit one dose of Kali. bich. 12C, to be repeated one week after that. Recommended also avoidance of dairy, wheat and sugar.

Three weeks later, phone conversation with her daughter: '...so much better...her old self...wonderful.'

Two weeks after this her daughter is in our office: 'still improving...she even went out shopping on her own which she had not done for approx. 5 months... and she is meticulously taking her remedies.'

One month after this follow-up she is still doing well, with winter approaching to raise her vital force/resistance two doses of Sulphur 30C one week apart, followed about seven weeks later by one weekly dose of Calc. carb. 12C as a longer term 'maintenance' in view of her own and also inherent heart predisposition.

She did indeed get through the winter more easily, her energy was fine, cataract seems not affected in either way, the belching began to noticeably improve with Calc. carb.

CASE 2

Female
Age: 40

EW had been suffering from depression for many years. A close friend had just committed suicide and she felt 'raw, exposed and hurt'. Her mother at age 44 committed suicide when EW was just 10 years of age. EW was married with two children. She was 5ft 10in tall and weighed 150lb. Her hair was light brown and her eyes brown.

Family History

Her father had a bad temper and was a hypochondriac. For example, he would often mistake indigestion for a heart attack. Her mother was an alcoholic and prescription drug abuser. She was also a hypochondriac and committed suicide at age 44. Her brother, John, died in a car accident three months later. Her brother Bill, aged 45, had a nervous breakdown. Her maternal grandfather was diabetic and her grandmother died of a heart attack in her early seventies. Her paternal grandfather died in a car accident before she was born and the grandmother died of leukaemia at age 83 (four out of five siblings died of some form of cancer).

Patient History

EW had appendicitis and an appendectomy at age 4. She had pneumonia at age 4 and again at age 7. She also had a tonsillectomy at 8 years of age.

Present Complaints

The patient's chief complaints were depression and grief. She was irritable, cried easily and was unable to think clearly. She had a 'foggy feeling'. She had been taking anti-depressive allopathic medicine for many years.

Mental Characteristics

EW had been depressed since her childhood after the death of her mother. She was especially 'filled with' the depression on Sundays and around major holidays, such as Thanksgiving or Christmas. She absolutely 'hated the holidays'. If things went well for her, she would 'wait for the other shoe to drop'. She was initially shy with people then would become sociable. She did not like to be the centre of attention with everybody. She felt ashamed if criticized. She was indecisive and then questioned her decisions after they were made. She was intuitive and felt insecure about love. She was a 'cold person but didn't like to be hot'.

Modalities

She was worse between 4 and 6pm. During the holidays and on Sundays she was more depressed than usual. She was tired from 2 to 3pm.

Physical Complaints

EW had a 20 per cent hearing loss in her right ear and a 10 per cent hearing loss in her left ear. She had a constant ringing in both ears. She was a hungry person and her thirst was 'so-so'. Her stools were 'loose' while she was taking Zoloft. Two years ago she had an abnormal smear. They excised it and the subsequent pap smear was normal. When she got a cold it usually settled in her chest and developed into bronchitis. She bathed frequently and consequently her skin was dry. She was nearsighted and had astigmatism. She clenched her teeth and chewed on her cheek. She had few fillings. When she experienced hay fever she had itchy eyes and sinus congestion. Her diet 'was not very good'; she craved sugar, fat and salt. She loved to sleep and slept well at night. She had constant, vivid, chaotic dreams and had snake dreams all her life. The snake dreams did not occur as often. She had aversions to snakes, heights, the dark, dying, leaving her children and strange men.

Prescription

Plussing Technique

Pulsatilla 30C hourly for one day then decrease to QID

August 1 There was an immediate effect when she started taking the Pulsatilla. She felt much better, was thinking clearer and was not so emotional. Prescription – continue Pulsatilla 30C

October 27 EW was starting 'to slip back'. The depression was not improving as well. Prescription – Pulsatilla 200C once per day

November 25 The holidays were going very well. It was the best Thanksgiving she had ever had. She felt 'real even'. She was looking forward to the Christmas holidays. She experienced some depression three days before her period. It stopped when the flow started. She also experienced some depression on Sundays. She had not had any colds and her dreams were more like 'everyday' dreams. Prescription – Continue Pulsatilla 200C treatment plan. Her menstrual cycle will begin in one week. I advised her to keep track of her symptoms of depression to see if there were any improvements or changes. We will meet again at that time and re-evaluate.

CASE 3

Miss G
Age: 15

Presenting Symptoms

Asthma attacks since October 1990, diagnosed as asthma by GP and hospital specialist. Started with a cold and occasional ear infection.

91

Hospitalized three times in October 1990. Eyes sore. Nose lacrimation profuse. Profuse sneezing for three days; on the fourth day a cough started. Discharge like white of an egg. Worse 1am, usually when attack starts. Better sitting up. Worse lying down. Better uncovered. Wheezing expectoration frothy. Usually settles back to sleep 3am. Skin – dry, rough in places.

Observations

Small, dark-haired, pale skin, slightly round-shouldered. Respiration fast. Polite and quiet for age. Fidgety and restless.

Allopathic Treatment

Ventalin Inhaler, three puffs twice a day, morning and night. Becatide 50, three puffs twice a day, morning and night.

Past History

Mother - fit and well
Father – slight eczema
Paternal mother/grandfather – not known
Maternal grandfather – not known
Maternal grandmother – bronchitis

Birth

Caesarean section, 7lb 6oz. Breech presentation. Occasional nappy rash and cradle cap. Breast fed. History of vomiting from birth to 7 months then settled. Childhood diseases – none. Coughs and colds.

Vaccinations

DPT 3 months. Measles

Mind

Afraid of worms.
Afraid of dark occasionally.
Likes attention – enjoys company, likes to be read to, enjoys drawing.
Can be sensitive.
Occasional nightmares.
Dislikes cream, vegetables, cream cakes and eggs. Poor appetite.
Likes fish and ice-cream. Likes milk every day. Likes cold and warm drinks.

Bowels

Regular every day

Urine

No problem

What Has to be Cured?

Asthma
STRATEGY: To treat the symptoms and miasm
METHOD: Classical
REMEDIES: Arsenicum 6C TDS three weeks plus Bach Flower Rescue Remedy for child and mother
JUSTIFICATION: Time worse 1 to 2am
ASTHMA: Wheezy, Profuse lacrimation, Restlessness,Better sitting up, Craves cold drinks, Fear of being alone, Expectoration frothy, Skin eruptions
Fever burning heat, Better uncovered
Expectations: Improve symptoms and reduce attacks
ADVICE: Discuss with GP regarding reduction of drugs. Mother very stressed at times of attacks, gently pointed this out to her and advised to take Rescue Remedy at the times of attacks. Felt that if the mother remained calm, the patient would benefit.

Discussed homoeopathy and printed information given.
Next appointment: 2 weeks
REASON: My practice is to see patients two weeks after the first prescription.

Second Visit 14/5/91

MOTHER STATES: Much better after starting remedy.
1 day sneezing, slight cough, no asthma attacks. Appetite and thirst the same.
Sleeping well, not so hot as before. Drugs: Becatide and Ventalin discussed with hospital specialist. More colour in the face. Skin better. Energy better.
Continue with Arsenicum, feel it is working.

Third Visit 3/6/91

Looks very well.
Started with a slight cold last week.
Runny nose for two days.
No asthma attack.
Complains of pain in left ear. I am mother called GP and put her on antibiotics. Child sick after first one, so did not give her any more.
Sleeping well. Hot at night. Appetite good. Craving milk. Lot of energy. Drugs: Becatide and Ventalin once a day. Skin now looks like goose pimples – much improved. Very chatty and more extrovert. Rosy red cheeks. Suddenly fastidious.
REMEDY: Tuberculinum 1M single dose
Arsenicum 6C
Belladonna 30C/200C. Given to the mother with advice to use
Ferrum phos. 6X, if required
(Nosode given, it is indicated by symptoms together with family history.)

Fourth Visit 6/8/91

No attack for two months.
Skin clear.
Only uses Ventalin occasionally when the mother thinks she is breathing and wheezing in the evenings.
Blocked nose – morning lasts two hours, better fresh air
Discharge – thick and yellow/green
Suddenly averse fat, butter and ice-cream
Dreams – couple of nightmares.
Urine and bowels – regular.

Justification of Prescription

Tuberculinum
Family miasm from maternal grandmother – bronchitis. Father's eczema. Child hyperactive. Flushed cheeks. Increased craving for milk. Night sweats. Ear infection. Habits changing suddenly, becoming fastidious. Chatty, extrovert.

Belladonna

In case Tuberculinum action produced a curative fever. Together with Ferrum phos. – for any inflammation.

Pulsatilla

Pulsatilla 30C TDS 1 week. Child was excited about starting school. Showed signs of clinging. Discharge yellow/green thick. Worse evening. Avoid fat, butter, ice-cream (which normally craved). Better fresh air. Thirst – less. Fear – night.

Fifth Visit 2/9/91

Mother states child happy and content.
Skin clear.
Chest clear.

Slight nasal discharge two days reduced on its own. Sleeps well, undisturbed.
Energy good ++

Appetite poor for two days but good now.

No prescription. See in six weeks. Feel Pulsatilla still working.

Sixth Visit 28/10/91

No colds, no coughs. Used to get a cold every other week with asthma symptoms, especially starting this month but none so far this season.

No tears. Happy and content at school. Settled well – no problems. Has made new friends.

Skin clear. Still on Ventalin – one puff daily.

No prescription.

Child to see specialist next week at hospital. Will discuss stopping Ventalin completely. Mother agreed.

Seventh Visit 2/12/91

Specialist discharged child with instructions to stop Ventalin within a week.

Mother says child is fine now.

Much better energy.

No problems at school. Lively, more outgoing and not shy.

Appetite – eating everything.

Thirst – increased (back to normal) drinking both hot and cold.

Bowels and urine regular.

Sleep – through night

Dreams – none.

No asthma, cough or colds. Has grown 2in.

No prescription. To contact me if any problems.

Check up in four months.

I believe these symptoms arose from grandmother's history of chest, father's skin conditions, together with suppressed cradle cap and nappy rash. All made worse by the fact that the patient is an only child of an overly protective mother.

Arsenicum started the cure. Tuberculinum completed the chest/asthma symptoms and Pulsatilla managed very well to put the child at ease and to adapt to change.

Repertory Kent

Rubrics used:

Visit 1

Frightened easily 49
Company desired for 12
Frightened waking on 49
Fear night alone 42
Desires cold drinks 484
Desires milk 485
Desires warm drinks 486
Appetite wanting 479
Averse fat and rich food 480
Cough wheezing asthmatic 782
Cough wheezing must sit up 803
Expectoration frothy 815
Cough after midnight 781
Sneezing 350
Sneezing frequent 351
Nose discharge copious 330
Skin dry 1307
REMEDY: Arsenicum 30C

Visit 3

Excitable 40
Fear night 42
Averse fats 480
Averse ice-cream – frozen foods   1363
Better fresh air 1344
Catarrh green, thick 331
Catarrh yellow/green 333
Worse evening 1342
REMEDY: Pulsatilla 30C

CASE 4

Female patient, Pauline
Age: 55
Divorced, three children (now 34 years, 31 years and 22 years)

Past history

Mastitis – 26 years ago.
Rheumatic fever.

Presenting symptoms

Pauline had a car accident in January. *Has never been well since* and experiences shifting pain all over her body. Stiffness in elbows and knees. She is often stressed and has had a series of accidents including falling downstairs.
Extreme tiredness – mental and physical. Lethargic. Suffering from mood swings and depression. Lacks interest in everything. Loss of appetite when fatigued.
Some memory loss. Vague thoughts leading to making mistakes.
Feels anxious that her health is deteriorating.
Frequent nauseous headaches – like a migraine lasting for several hours. 'Cannot shake it off.' Sweats.
Feels lightheaded and sometimes has difficulty focusing her eyes.
Irritation in rectum with alternating constipation and diarrhoea.
Legs often ache with some numbness.
Distended abdomen with flatulence.

Modalities

Worse sitting. Worse in spring. Better hot drinks.

Constitution

Pauline has dark hair with blue eyes, slim, pale complexion, 5ft 6in tall, weighing 8st 2lb (constant over last 4 months).

Prescription

Bacillus No 7, 30C one dose (two tablets)
Lithium carb., 6C one dose daily

She is very positive. Always wants to do things even though she lacks the energy. Violent mood swings – manic depression. A goal setter who is a workaholic. She 'does not suffer fools gladly'. Punctual. Very tidy and organized. Creative with artistic flair. Often feels frustrated. Domineering. Bouts of anxiety. Likes wine and smokes 'a few' cigarettes each day.

25 May 1995

Feels less tired.
Appetite has improved.
Still sweats a little.
Only one headache since first consultation.
Still suffering mood swings.
Some stiffness in limbs.
Prescription: Lithium carb. 6C twice daily between meals

6 November 1995

She feels 'much more stabilized'.
Fewer bouts of depression.
Occasional headaches.
Feeling more relaxed and more energetic.
Appetite good – eats a little often.
Less flatulence and abdomen 'less bloated'.

12 April 1996

Cheerful and has not been depressed 'since Christmas'.
Much less fatigued.
Memory much improved.

95

Now keeping very busy.
Moves with alacrity – little stiffness in limbs.
Still sweats occasionally, but not profusely.
Prescription: Continue dosing with
Lithium carb. 6C

2 June 1996

Her condition is still satisfactory. Progressing
well. No depression.
Prescription: Bacillus No 7 30C. Repeat
one dose

CASE 5
Female, Pamela
Age: 49 years
1st consultation 1.12.97
Divorced, no children

Occupation

Careline operator for four years.

Family

Mother – cervical cancer. 'Struggles' to care
for her mother.
Father – deceased (Stroke).
Both sisters menopausal problems.

Presenting symptoms

Loss of voice since 1 week before.
Catarrh for 2 weeks. Loose, bright yellow,
lumpy sputum.
Headaches on waking. Left temple.
Lacking energy.

Constitution

Light brown hair, pale complexion,
blue/green eyes. Weight constant over 6
months (9st 4lb). Prefers to be alone. Very

punctual. Anxiety frequent. Job is often
stressful. Likes travel. Hot feeling at times.

Modalities

< movement < warmth > morning > night

Prescription

Kali. bich. 30C, two tablets three times daily
between meals.

23 January 1998

Pamela reports that catarrh cleared over
Christmas.
Sore throat. Mouth ulcers on left side.
Suppuration. Slight inflammation in throat.
Prescription: Merc. Sol. 6C. Two tablets
three times daily with clean mouth.

3 February 1998

Pamela reports a marginal improvement in
the first few days only. Sore throat cleared.
Prescription: Hepar. Sulph. 6C. Two
tablets three times daily.

3 March 1998

Mouth ulcers completely cleared.
Stopped dosing.

CASE 6

Male, Surjit
Age: 15 years
First consultation 10.6.98

Surjit was of Indian parents, born in the UK.
He was quite robust, intelligent with a
friendly smile. He was wearing woollen
mittens even though it was a warm day.

He had suffered from eczema as an infant, like his father. Both parents in good health.

Present Complaint

Surjit was suffering from at least fifteen open 'cauliflower' type warts on the backs of both hands and fingers and between the fingers. The largest measured 8mm in diameter down to several the size of a pinhead.

The warts were painful, particularly when brushed by clothing, sometimes with slight bleeding. He was wearing the mittens not only to avoid painful abrasion, but also to prevent some warts between his fingers impingeing on one another and to avoid the embarrassment he experienced with his school friends at a particularly sensitive age.

He had suffered from these warts for about seven years. Conventional treatment had failed. In all other respects he was fit and healthy. There were no other skin problems.

PRESCRIPTION

Thuja 6C, two tablets orally three times daily between meals.
Thuja mother tincture, applied liberally, toplically, to saturate each individual wart three times a day and at night.

17.7.98

Considerable improvement on both hands. Some of the smaller warts had virtually disappeared and larger warts had decreased in size and appeared flatter and less eruptive.

PRESCRIPTION: Repeat of the original.

Surjit wore light cotton gloves after treating the warts. These were soothing and assisted the entrapment of the Thuja tincture in and around the warts.

25.8.98

Further significant diminution in size and a smoother appearance of some warts.

PRESCRIPTION: Acidum nitricum 6C, two tablets orally three times daily between meals. Acidum nitricum 5X, applied liberally to remaining warts three times daily.
Note: A potency lower than 5X of nitric acid was considered to run the risk of burning the skin.

16.11.98

The warts were almost completely healed. Apart from two or three which were slightly mounded, the only evidence of the remainder was slightly pink, new healthy, smooth skin.

PRESCRIPTION. Thuja mother tincture, applied to few remaining traces of the warts three times daily.

3.4.99

Surjit's hands were virtually clear of warts with two small, smooth mounded warts and only smooth flat new skin where warts were originally located, after seven years of pain, discomfort and embarrassment.

CASE 7

George
Age: 43 years
Two children aged 19 and 17 years
Occupation: Steel worker

History

George's wife had died suddenly following a stroke. He was informed when he arrived at the hospital. They had been married twenty-two years and he adored her. A month later when he was seeking treatment he was still stricken with grief and had not come to terms with her loss. He was sleeping badly and on waking he felt 'washed out' and 'more tired than when he went to bed', and felt weak and fatigued. He had sometimes sat up in bed about 2am feeling wide awake.

George and his wife kept themselves 'very much to themselves' during their married life. He was always better when alone or with his wife as he was basically a shy person, avoided crowds and liked peace and quiet. He could not return to work.

He blamed himself to some extent for his wife's death as he thought he could have done more to help her in the house so she could have rested more. He thought her stroke was brought on by 'overdoing it'. He thought perhaps that he had sometimes fussed over things that were not important.

George was dark-haired with brown eyes. A timid, gentle, sensitive person of a nervous temperament who liked an orderly routine and worried about little things. He was happier alone or with his children and found it difficult to relax with strangers.

He did not smoke (hates tobacco smell) and drank one cup of coffee a day.

Repertorization

By computer over 15 rubrics indicated Ignatia closely followed by Natrum mur.

PRESCRIPTION: Ignatia 200, three pilules every second day

Three weeks later patient was feeling more relaxed and containing his grief. Feeling slightly less exhausted. Occasional headaches.

PRESCRIPTION: Ignatia 1M, three pilules twice weekly

Six weeks later George was feeling much better, was visiting his children and had returned to work, although he found it difficult.

PRESCRIPTION: Ignatia 10M, one dose

CASE 8

On 20 May, I was taken to a cancer research hospital in Bombay to see Mr MH, aged 55, who was diagnosed as a case of Ca base of the tongue with secondaries in right pyriform fossa. He had developed severe cough, dyspnoea and fever. Chest X-ray showed cavitated lesion in the right mid-zone with air-fluid level. This was suggestive of abscess formation. A stony, hard, irregular, fixed, immovable mass measuring 2.5 to 3in in diameter was felt in the right side of the neck.

The hospital authorities had given up hope and my friend wanted to know whether homoeopathy would be able to help him.

When I visited him at his home, as the patient could not speak, most of the history was obtained from the wife and the relatives. In November he developed hoarseness of voice, cough and breathlessness which gradually increased. He was treated by several general practitioners without significant relief. Ultimately he was referred to the cancer research hospital. He gave past history of double pneumonia, typhoid and amoebic dysentery. A cyst was surgically removed which he had on his forehead. He suffered from boils off and on in the past. There was no significant family history. Aversions to sweet, salty food and milk. Tendency to flatulence – better passing flatus. Profuse perspiration on forehead when eating. Sleeps with legs elevated. Addicted to tea – eight to ten cups per day.

Used to smoke about thirty cigarettes per

day but stopped smoking since April. Highly irritable by nature, a man with self-respect who cannot bear injustice, brooding, symp-athetic and tendency to weep when emotional.

On back-checking the dates with the lunar calendar it was found that the time when he developed hoarseness of voice in November was just before full moon day. When I visited him in the cancer hospital on 20 May, it was also twelfth day of the lunar calendar. He was a little better thereafter when the hospital authorities discharged him at his request.

PRESCRIPTION: He was given Staphysagria 30C tds on the following indications on 1 June

1. Ailments from suppressed anger.
2. Tendency to suppuration.
3. Agg. before full moon.
4. Aversion to milk.

The cough and the breathlessness subsided in a week. His irritability of mind also reduced to a great extent and he gradually started improving. His appetite increased and he gained weight. He could swallow semi-solid food which he could not swallow before.

CASE 9

Attributed to Dr Nash (1936)
Female
Age: 40 years

Presenting Symptoms

Stiff neck of long standing. Severe pains and swellings of all finger joints. Pregnant for seven months. Sleeplessness through pain. Relief from covering fingers in mustard.

PRESCRIPTION: Caulophyllum 3X, three times daily. Pain in fingers was relieved but brought on labour pains.
Remedy discontinued for fear of premature labour (see Chapter 8).

Finger pain returned and continued until her baby was born.
Lochia, instead of decreasing, increased until it amounted to a metrorrhagia. Flow was passive, dark and fluid. Great sense of weakness. Internal trembling. Return of finger pain.

PRESCRIPTION: Arnica, Sabina, Secale, Sulphur.
No improvement.
Note: Caulophyllum, although indicated, was not prescribed for fear of bringing on bearing-down pains.

PRESCRIPTION: Caulophyllum 200C.
Patient completely cured, no pain. Did not return.

Nash added that in cases of small joints in hands and feet, as in rheumatoid arthritis in women, Caulophyllum must be considered. It had often regulated labour pains and in problems of the uterus and small joints during the menopause.

He was also convinced that had he prescribed Caulophyllum at the higher potency in the first instance, there would have been no problem.

CASE 10

Date: 23 July
Male
Age: 38

History

Client was suffering from insomnia and occasional episodes of shortness/tightness of the chest. He was 6ft 3in tall, weighing 180lb.

He was very friendly and ready to discuss his symptoms. However, he was fidgety during the consultation. His occupation was video producer over the last sixteen years. He and a partner managed their own company. He was extremely dedicated to his work and worked at times eighty to one hundred hours per week. He was a workaholic, overachiever and perfectionist. He had high expectations of himself and at times 'flew off the handle' because some of his clients frustrated him. He was very sensitive to noise/sounds and became very irritable if he was disturbed while working. He felt that his small town did not allow him to truly develop his talents.

His father had ulcers and his mother high blood pressure. He had no major illnesses. His insomnia began eleven months ago. He was very 'stressed out from work'. He went to bed at 9.30pm, read for half an hour, and then lay down to fall asleep. Shortly afterwards, he would wake up startled. He would read again until his 'eyes got tired' and often could not sleep because he would think of his work. He consistently woke up at 3.45am and it was difficult to go back to sleep. In the morning he was tired and unrefreshed and drank coffee to get started.

His episodes of shortness/tightness of the chest started four weeks ago. His respiration worsened and his heart pounded. It was worse with coffee and stress.

He experienced occasional headaches in the morning, which improved with coffee. He ate fast foods and especially liked the fatty foods, french fries and Pepsi. When he had hay fever, he experienced red itchy eyes, congested sinuses and postnasal drip. He also at times suffered from canker sores and herpes simplex, all aggravated by stress.

Prescription

Nux vomica 30C, three granules under tongue QID.

August 5

Generally, he was much calmer and not so anxious. He no longer experienced episodes of tightness in the chest. He was sleeping steadily from 10.30pm to 5.30am until a few days ago when his sleep became restless again. There were no hay fever symptoms.

PRESCRIPTION: Nux vomica 200C once per day in the morning.

August 30

The client 'felt better overall'. He still did not experience any episodes of tightness in the chest or hay fever. His sleep was much better and he slept consistently through the night until recently. He was under much more stress and started to wake up at 4am again.

PRESCRIPTION: Nux vomica 1M once per week.

September 24

Although client was under another 'high stress situation again', his insomnia was much better. It doesn't take him too long to fall asleep and he is not waking up in the middle of the night. Occasionally, he sleeps until 4.30am and then goes back to sleep until morning. There are no episodes of tightness in the chest and shortness of breath.

PRESCRIPTION: Continue Nux vomica 1M once per week until no further improvement.
Final dose of Nux vomica 10M.

CHAPTER 7
New Aspects of Homoeopathy

Homoeopathic research. Malaria: prophylaxis and homoeopathic treatment. Potency selection. Homoeopathy – art or science? Twelve new cell salts. Observations on the Doctrine of Signatures. Stimulation of the immune system. Bowel nosodes – a postscript. The nature of Causticum. Healing venoms.

RESEARCH INTO HOMOEOPATHY

Homoeopathy is a challenging, dynamic and flexible therapy, and to adopt a narrow, dogmatic and inflexible view is to deny it reaching its true potential.

Even though the Similimum is at its core, homoeopathy must not become a monolithic therapy if its growth is to continue in the twenty-first century. We must keep pace with the progress of medical and scientific knowledge if we are to avoid another decline. The homoeopathic book was not closed following the death of Hahnemann, nor even Kent. Like every modern discipline, homoeopathy needs research into its every facet and every homoeopath must play his or her part.

In this chapter I will look at some of my observations and research over twenty-five years in homoeopathy which I trust will prove to be a modest contribution in advancing our understanding of the Healing Art.

MALARIA: PROPHYLAXIS AND ITS HOMOEOPATHIC TREATMENT

This account is based on a paper presented at the Liga Congress in Amsterdam, April 1998.

Introduction

The widespread use, about twenty-five years ago, of the pesticide DDT, which kills the mosquito parasitic protozoa responsible for spreading malaria, led scientists to believe the disease would be completely eradicated. However, during the 1970s most countries ceased to use DDT when it was found to be highly toxic to animals and wildlife. As a result there has been an upsurge in the mosquito population and the incidence of malaria has now reached alarming proportions. The World Health Organization estimates that malaria now affects up to five hundred million people world-wide, killing about two million children each year. Additionally, drug-resistant strains of the disease parasites have developed in recent years. Resistance to most allopathic drugs, including quinine, is now increasing inexorably and the allopathic drug companies are urgently seeking new drugs to stem the tide.

Malarial Cycle

The parasitic protozoa of the genus plasmodia are responsible for the disease. They are transmitted by the bite of an infected female Anopheles mosquito. Only four of the hundred species of these protozoa are responsible for infecting humans, falciparum, virax, malariae and ovale. The parasites enter the body in the saliva of the female when they are carried to the liver. A cascade of asexual multiplication of the parasites in the liver cells cause the symptoms of malaria, which include shivers with rising temperature followed by fever, intense sweating, headache, nausea, dizziness and vomiting.

As homoeopaths, we are reminded of Hahnemann's original experiment with Cinchona (Peruvian bark) in Stotteritz in 1791, when he reported the symptoms he experienced after taking 'four drams of China twice daily', as being similar to those of 'intermittent fever [malaria], palpitations, intolerable anxiety, trembling, prostration in all the limbs, redness of cheeks, quick and hard pulse, pulsation in the head and thirst'.

Allopathic Treatment of Malaria

Quinine, the principal constituent of Cinchona (8 per cent), was isolated by the allopaths as 4-quinoline methanol in 1820; the indigenous people of South America being the first to use the natural infusion of the bark. This bitter-tasting alkaloid has been used extensively in its synthetic form all over the world for the treatment of malaria and proved to be very effective. In recent years, however, the spread of resistance to the drug has restricted its use to limited areas, such as Central America. In Thailand, Cambodia and Vietnam the problem is causing major alarm. It is feared that resistance to quinine will spread to Africa, where 90 per cent of fatalities from malaria occur.

This potentially disastrous situation led to the search by allopaths for similar, more effective drugs. Chloroquinine, pyrimethamine and now mefloquine (sold as Larium) have all been tried but resistance to them is increasing all the time. Additionally Lariam, although ten times as potent as quinine and shown to work effectively against chloroquinine-resistant parasites, has been condemned by the media as having alleged serious side-effects, including seizures, epileptic fits and manic depression. However, the UK Department of Health believes that the risks associated with Lariam are extremely low.

Homoeopathic Treatment of Malaria

Cinchona officinalis (China) in potency has traditionally been prescribed for the homoeopathic treatment of malarial symptoms and in the 30th centesimal potency in a daily dose as a prophylactic. Other remedies prescribed, to a lesser extent, are principally Ipecacuanha, Coffea, Galeum and Mitchella, all of which are of the same natural order of plants as Cinchona itself (Rubiaceae), and Chinium sulphuricum (quinine sulphate), and Chinium muriaticum (quinine chloride). Notwithstanding the power of the Similimum, in view of the increasing ineffectiveness of synthetic quinine against malarial symptoms, no doubt exacerbated by the allopathic macromolecular dosages employed (about 0.05g), arguably we must consider the present status of efficacy of homoeopathic potencies of Cinchona and associated remedies.

Scientists know that quinine works by concentrating in the digestive vacuole of the malarial parasite and inhibiting the availability of iron by forming a complex compound of iron – porphyrin – which is toxic to the parasite.

Dr V.A. Van Erp and Dr Martin Brands published a paper in the British Homoeopathic Journal, Vol. 95, pp. 66–70 in April 1996. They reported that in Tamale in Ghana 40 per cent of the population is infected with the plasmodium parasite.

They conducted a pilot study and a short double blind clinical trial. Inclusion and exclusion criteria were specified but for ethical reasons no placebo was employed. A single dose tailored to each individual patient was given at 30C potency and around twenty homoeopathic remedies were used. The other half were given chloroquine.

Improvement according to pre-defined criteria was 72 per cent in the chloroquine group and 83 per cent in the homoeopathy group. However, the difference was not statistically significant and the authors recognized the increasing drug resistance of the plasmodium parasite and an alternative treatment would be a major breakthrough.

Since 1992 research has been concentrated on the alkaloid Artemisinin (8-hydroxysantonin), which has also been shown to reduce the availability of iron to the malarial parasite, but much more effectively than quinine.

In 1996 a research team at Johns Hopkins University, Baltimore, US, reported their findings on artemisinin extracts from the buds of the sweet-scented flowers of the shrub Artemisia annua.

Conclusion

There are twenty-five different plant sub-species of Artemisia (Compositae), of which Artemisia abrotanum (Abrotanum),

Artemisia maritima (Cina), Artemisia absinthium (Absinthium) are fully proved homoeopathic remedies, listed in all the homoeopathic *Materia Medicas*. Their proving symptoms embrace those associated with Cinchona officinalis and suggest that these remedies should be studied in relation to future homoeopathic treatment of malarial symptoms as a matter of some urgency.

With Artemisia vulgaris, for example, we have proving symptoms, inter alia, of fever with profuse sweating, drowsiness, stupor, dizziness, shooting pains in the head, trembling, fatigue in lower limbs, nausea and vomiting. Apart from the *Materia Medicas*, the remedy receives scant attention in the classic homoeopathic textbooks, so it now behoves us to take a closer look in the context of malarial treatment and prophylaxis.

I have communicated with Professor Gary Posner and his team in Baltimore with a view to the study of our proved homoeopathic remedies prepared from mother tinctures of sub-species of the Artemisia plant family. Although their approach is allopathic, nevertheless their scientific findings are valuable in homoeopathic studies.

HAHNEMANN POTENCIES

Samuel Hahnemann never prescribed in potencies higher than the 30th centesimal potency. Later in his life he experimented with 60C, but never higher.

His original choice of potency numbers were 3, 6, 12, 24, 30 (and later 60), in both decimal and centesimal potencies. I was taught that these potencies are favoured even today because they generally correspond to levels of optimum therapeutic efficacy. There is some confirmation of this explanation given by research carried out by Doctor Jones and Doctor Jenkins at the Royal London Homoeopathic Hospital in 1981, studying wheat and yeast growth rates stimulated by different potencies. The work followed similar studies by Doctor Pelikan and Doctor Unger with potencies of Argentum nitricum (1971). Using centesimal potencies of Argentum nitricum, Arnica montana and several other remedies, increasing mean extension growth rates were observed with increasing potencies and peak growth rates roughly coincided with those chosen by Hahnemann.

However, I questioned why Hahnemann had chosen these potencies in the first place. He had no research or clinical data to guide him so he must have chosen these numbers

as 'benchmarks' for testing the effectiveness of his new-found therapy, and building up his own clinical experience.

It was clear to me that he was influenced by the common numerical system used in everyday life in Europe in the nineteenth century. This old system – the *duodecimal* system – was based on units, sub-units or multiples of the number 12. Hence Hahnemann chose 3, 6, 12, 24, 30, 60. This observation is now sometimes kindly referred to as *Cook's hypothesis*.

At that time, the Saxon coinage was based on the 'Friedrichs D'or', a gold coin that was divided into twelve units called 'thalers'. Many other examples of the duodecimal system still remain today: for example, there are twelve hours on the clock face, twelve

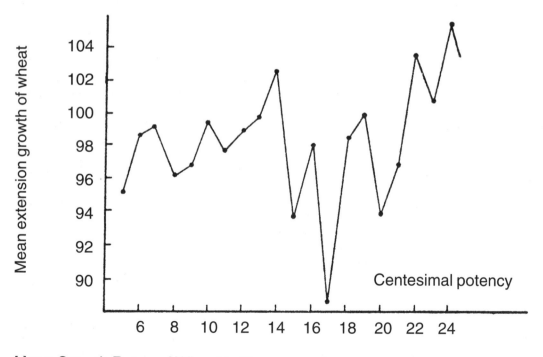

Mean Growth Rates of Wheat in Presence of
Centesimal Potencies of Arnica

inches to one foot and, until 1969, twelve old pence equalled one shilling.

Once again, Hahnemann displayed an uncanny foresight in establishing homoeopathy in choosing these potencies that are those most frequently prescribed even today. I suggest that a study of the efficacy of potencies representing an extrapolation of these potency numbers, that is 36, 42, 48, 72 etc., would be useful.

It might be argued, however, that if my hypothesis is correct, then why are commonly prescribed higher potencies based on the *metric* or *decimal* system, based in units, sub-units or multiples of 10? These are 200, 1,000(1M), 10,000 (10M), 50,000(50M) and 100,000(CM).

The explanation must lie with the fact that these high potencies were introduced into homoeopathic practice about seventy years later following the teachings of Dr James Tyler Kent *et al.* By this time the metric system had been widely adopted in the learned fields of medicine and science so it would have seemed logical for Kent and his associates to adopt metric or decimal units when introducing these higher potencies into practice.

HOMOEOPATHY – ART OR SCIENCE?

Another question I have considered is why did Hahnemann use the duodecimal system of numbering in choosing the potencies he would *prescribe* when he had used the decimal system for the *preparation* of homoeopathic remedies? Thus we have:

Decimal series of potencies dilution ratio 1:10
Centesimal series of potencies dilution ratio 1:100
The answer surely lies in the fact that while

Hahnemann described in his writings the method for the preparation of potencies as an exact science, the actual practice of homoeopathy was an art. The original title for his quintessential work was 'The Organon of the Healing **Art**'.

Hahnemann was also a scientist. He studied chemistry at the University of Leipzig and, even at that time, in the late eighteenth century, the scientists and men of learning used the decimal or metric system in their work. It is logical then that Hahnemann would use this system in his scientific work.

CELL SALTS

The original twelve cell salts of the German physician W.H. Schüssler are commonly regarded as the homoeopathic equivalent of mineral and vitamin supplementation. The twelve cell salts (tissue salts or biochemic remedies) are fully proved homeopathic remedies and as such their curative action is employed in the classical Hahnemannian manner. Boericke and Dewey likened the action of these biochemic remedies of Schüssler to 'the opposite blade of the scissors'.

In 1846, Constantine Hering wrote in Stapf's Archives that 'all constituents of the human body principally act on those organs wherein they have a function. All fulfil their functions when they are the cause of symptoms', thus foreshadowing Dr Schüssler's new biochemic theory.

It was not until 1873 that Dr Schüssler introduced his 'new biochemic system' whereby he claimed that his biochemic remedies acted by correcting inorganic mineral nutritional deficiencies. He claimed that his system was in no way related to the homoeopathic Law of Similars, but upon physiological–chemical processes in the organism. However, when it was pointed out that the twelve cell salts were already included in the homoeopathic *Materia Medica*, he later conceded the relationship. Nevertheless, Schüssler's work opened up and renewed interest in these remedies and fuller provings which raised them to the status of near polycrests.

Biochemic cell salts, or tissue salts, are now stocked in low potencies by pharmacies and health food stores world-wide and enjoy a popularity with lay people both as sources of essential nutrients and homoeopathic self-treatment. Thousands of people have followed up this simple, readily available introduction to homoeopathy with seeking treatment by homoeopathic physicians for more serious conditions.

Schüssler's biochemical theory

Schüssler recognized that organic substances were vital to the human organism, but he believed that they cannot perform their proper functions without mineral inorganic substances.

The functions of these essential minerals in the body are now understood to act as components of enzymes essential for nerve impulse transmission, the formation of building blocks for bones and teeth and as components of hormones.

The biochemic theory of Dr Schüssler may be summarized simply as follows:

1. The human body contains twelve vital inorganic substances that are responsible for the maintenance of normal cell function.
2. When from some cause, one or more of these substances become deficient the normal cell function or metabolism is disturbed and a condition arises known as disease.

Schüssler's Original Twelve Cell Salts

Common name	Latin name	Formula
1. Calcium fluoride	Calcarea fluorica	CaF_2
2. Calcium phosphate	Calcarea phosphorica	$Ca_3(PO_4)_2$
3. Calcium sulphate	Calcarea sulphurica	$CaSO_4$
4. Iron phosphate	Ferrum phosphorica	$Fe_3(PO_4)_2$
5. Potassium chloride	Kalium muriaticum	KCl
6. Potassium phosphate	Kalium phosphorica	K_3PO_4
7. Potassium sulphate	Kalium sulphuricum	K_2SO_4
8. Magnesium phosphate	Magnesia phosphorica	$Mg_3(PO_4)_2$
9. Sodium chloride	Natrum muriaticum	$NaCl$
10. Sodium phosphate	Natrum phosphoricum	Na_3PO_4
11. Sodium sulphate	Natrum sulphuricum	Na_2SO_4
12. Silicon dioxide	Silicea	SiO_2

3. By supplying the system of deficient elements (or nutrients) in the form of biochemic remedies (or cell salts or tissue salts), normal cell function and health are restored.

These inorganic mineral element nutrients were identified in Schüssler's time as:

Calcium	Ca	metal
Phosphorus	P	non-metal
Magnesium	Mg	metal
Iron	Fe	metal
Sodium	Na	metal
Potassium	K	metal
Fluorine	F	non-metal
Sulphur	S	non-metal
Chlorine	Cl	non-metal
Silicon	Si	non-metal

Schüssler introduced his twelve cell salts, which were all inorganic salts selected to embrace all the essential nutrients known to chemistry and medicine at that time. He presented them as essential for the proper growth and development of every part of the body's system. The salts were numbered 1 to 12 for ease of identification.

Modern Nutritional Knowledge

As previously explained, Schüssler's choice of the original cell salts was confined to the essential mineral nutrients known at the time (1873). Since then great strides have been made in nutritional research and our understanding of the functions of the healthy organism. Other nutrients have since been identified as key factors in the maintenance of good health. These minerals, required in the diet in very small quantities, are termed trace elements or micro nutrients. Deficiencies of these essential nutrients in the diet can have a profound

effect on the entire organism, which may be cataclysmic.

These trace elements or micro nutrients are listed below, with the year of those most recently identified as essential nutrients* shown.

Chromium	Cr	Metal
Manganese	Mn	Metal
Selenium	Se	Metalloid
Copper	Cu	Metal
Cobalt	Co	Metal
Zinc	Zn	Metal
Iodine	I	Non-metal
Lithium(1955)	Li	Metal
Boron(1981)	B	Metalloid
Molybdenum (1983)	Mo	Metal
Vanadium (1985)	V	Metal

*Aluminium, arsenic, cadmium, germanium, lead, nickel and tin are trace elements also identified in the human metabolism, but their biological value is only vaguely understood and some are toxic.

In 1993 the author carefully studied all mineral remedies in the homoeopathic *Materia Medica* which contain one or more of these new elements recently identified as essential nutrients among their constituents.

In every case, disorders arising in the human organism resulting from a dietary deficiency of these elements matched the key proving symptoms of the remedy.

The Twelve New Cell Salts

My thesis, therefore, is that any fully proved homoeopathic remedy that contains one or more of the essential mineral nutrients not known to Schüssler has the potential to act as a cell salt conforming with the biochemical theory. I have been selective in choosing those remedies whose criteria suggest optimum clinical efficacy in this context. For example, it should be noted that, where possible, the nutrients presented in the form of a mineral salt rather than the elements themselves are preferred. The ionized atoms of these elements (M^{n+} or X^{n-}) can enter into spontaneous combin-ation to form electrovalent bonds with other atoms, thus rendering the elements biologically available more readily.

The author proposed the following 'new' cell salts to be added to those of Schüssler. I must emphasize that their inclusion is in no way counter to Schüssler's theory nor to classical homoeopathic principles. All the remedies are listed in the homoeopathic *Materia Medica* and are fully proven.

Below are some examples.

Remedy: *CUPRUM ACETICUM (COPPER ACETATE)*

Nutritional properties of copper
Copper deficiency results in anaemia (necessary with iron for the formation of haemoglobin), diarrhoea, speech defects, muscle spasms, cramp, rigidity and neurotic brain behaviour, weight loss, exhaustion.

Proving symptoms of the remedy
MIND: Decreased brain functions. Delirium. Maniacal talking. Use of unintentional words. Loss of consciousness. Convulsions. Fatigue.
HEAD: Vertigo. Brain inflammation. Violent, throbbing headache.
STOMACH: Diarrhoea. Colic. Vomiting (green/white). Weight loss.
EXTREMITIES: Drawing and tension in all limbs. Numbness. Cramp in calves. Spasmodic contractions of fingers and toes. Stiffness of limbs. Paralysis.
The relationship between the proving symptoms of the homoeopathic remedy and

the metabolic role of the essential mineral nutrient contained therein is clear if we compare them.

Remedy: *LITHIUM CARBONICUM (LITHIUM CARBONATE*

Nutritional properties of lithium
Deficiency of lithium in dietary intake affects the entire organism. Mood swings. Manic depressive illness. Chronic rheumatism. Stiffness in limbs.
Excess of lithium interferes with thyroid function – insomnia, weight loss, weakness.

Proving symptoms of the remedy
MIND: Depression. Moodiness. Anxiety (< morning). Nightmares. Lethargy.
HEAD: Headaches. Confusion. Dizziness. Head feels large.
ABDOMEN: Pain in right kidney. Burning in urethra. Sore bladder. Stools light yellow.
EXTREMITIES: Rheumatic pain in small joints, particularly lower limbs. Swelling in small joints. Paralytic stiffness in all limbs.
SKIN: Body rash. Itching.

All symptoms:
< morning < right side < pressure movement.

Thus, by the same argument, relating proving symptoms and the symptoms arising from the deficiency or excess of the nutrient contained in the remedy, we can draw up the twelve new cell salts, all drawn from the *Materia Medica*:

1 CUPRUM ACETICUM, Copper acetate, $Cu(CH_3CO_2)_2$
2. LITHIUM CARBONICUM, Lithium carbonate, Li_2CO_3
3. COBALTUM METALLICUM,Cobalt metal, Co
4. SELENIUM, Selenium, Se

5. CHROMIUM OXIDATUM, Chromic oxide, Cr_2O_3
6. ZINC SULPHURICUM, Zinc sulphate, $ZnSO_4$
7. MANGANUM ACETICUM, Manganese acetate, $Mn(CH_3CO_2)_2$
8. IODUM, Iodine , I
9. VANADIUM, Vanadium metal, V
10. MANGANUM MURIATICUM, Manganese chloride, $MnCl_2$
11. ZINCUM METALLICUM, Zinc metal, Zn
12. BORAX, Sodium borate, $Na_2B_4O_7$

Potency

Whereas Schüssler recommended dosing of his original tissue salts at 3X or 6X potencies, the infinitesimally small nutritional levels required of the 'new' minerals in micrograms call for dosing at 6C or 12X potencies.

THE DOCTRINE OF SIGNATURES

Although it has no scientific basis, the Doctrine of Signatures, involving study of the intrinsic properties of natural substances in order to provide pointers to their

Linking of layers of carbon atoms in Graphites

Surface layers of skin cells

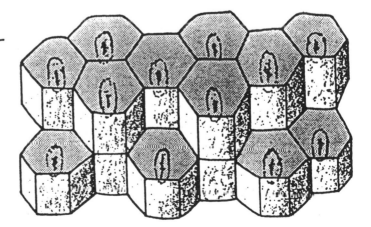

109

therapeutic value, has enjoyed a revival of interest in recent years.

For all its subjectivity, it does remind us, as homoeopaths, that homoeopathy is a natural holistic therapy. Our roots are in nature and we become too mechanistic at our peril. Hahnemann himself believed that 'nature has provided the means for mankind to cure all its ills and it is for man to seek out those means'.

I remember a homoeopathic practitioner being asked the source of the remedy, Bufo, to which he replied, 'I think it comes from some sort of plant'!

I have studied many plant sources of remedies and examples of the doctrine are relatively easy to find. The appearance, shape, flowers, growth patterns, habitats and other botanical features of plants all present therapeutic indictors which homoeopathic provings invariably confirm.

However, inanimate substances present less obvious features. The remedy Graphites is prepared from the soft, natural, chemically inactive allotropic form of the element, Carbon. It is recognized as a great antipsoric remedy. Its affinity with human skin indicated by the Doctrine of Signatures seemed a daunting prospect.

The element graphite has a crystalline structure based on layers of carbon atoms arranged in regular (six-sided) hexagons. It is the sliding of these layers or sheets of carbon atoms on one another that give graphite the smooth, slippery sensation when rubbed with the fingers.

The author noted a remarkable correlation between this crystalline structure and the arrangement of skin cells in the epithelium. The outer skin cells are arranged in a cuboidal and columnar structure which compares closely with the hexagonal graphite structure (see diagram).

Yet another example where one might be about to abandon the Doctrine of Signatures

as allegorical or metaphorical but then pause to reconsider.

THE BOWEL NOSODES: ASSOCIATED REMEDIES

Our working knowledge of the bowel nosodes is drawn primarily from a lecture by Dr John Paterson given at the meeting of the Liga Homeopatica Internationale in France in 1949 and its subsequent publication entitled 'The Bowel Nosodes', published in the British Homoeopathic Journal of July 1950. The original paper was published in the British Homoeopathic Journal in 1936 under the title 'The Potentized Drug and its Action on the Bowel Flora'.

The list of remedies representative of and associated with the bowel nosode, Sycotic Co., given by Paterson includes *Calcarea metallicum* (calcium metal). Allen's 'Keynotes with Nosodes' also lists *Calcarea metallicum*, but this is almost certainly a copy of Paterson's paper.

The list was amended in September 1949 and a mistake could have crept in here, as a search of a range of homoeopathic *Materia Medicas*, including Boericke, Clarke, Faringdon etc. and a computer scan does not include Calcarea metallicum as a remedy. This apparent omission led me to study this 'remedy' more closely.

The author assumed that the remedy Paterson had in mind was, in fact, *Calcarea caustica* (calcarea causticum), since the chemistry of the element, calcium, is such that a mother tincture (and hence potencies) of calcium metal is impossible to prepare. Calcarea caustica is a common remedy originally proved by Koch and is listed in all the standard *Materia Medicas*. Calcium metal reacts spontaneously with water (with a risk of fire!) to form the compound calcium hydroxide, formula $Ca(OH)_2$ (calcarea causticum).

110

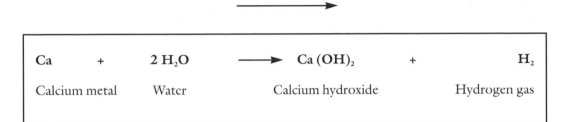

Ca	+	2 H₂O	⟶	Ca (OH)₂	+	H₂
Calcium metal		Water		Calcium hydroxide		Hydrogen gas

If we study the drug picture of Calc. caust., we see that its proving symptoms are dominated by profuse mucus, undoubtedly associated with irritation of the mucous membranes which, of course, is the keynote (gonorrheal) of Sycotic Co. We also find excessive mucus in nose and throat with nausea and vomiting and mucus in the stool. There are also skin problems including rashes. Undoubtedly, Calc. caust. is an associated remedy of Sycotic Co.

The author is convinced, therefore, that Bach and Paterson really thought of Calc. met. and Calc. caust. as synonymous. After all, as stated, Calc. caust. is simply the element calcium metal 'dissolved' in water (and alcohol).

In the light of the above, the author suggests that Dr Paterson's original paper should now be amended accordingly.

IMMUNE SYSTEM STUDIES

During the late 1970s and into the 1980s, the identification of a whole range of chemical substances produced by the body's immune system advanced our understanding of its natural defence mechanism against disease.

The first of these substances was *Interferon*, an organic polypeptide produced in human blood cells in response to an invasive disease virus, whence it passes into the plasma and counters the virus. A number of other Interferon derivatives, followed by a range of *Interleukins*, have since been identified and research is continuing. This demonstration of the body's natural defence mechanism is, of course, compatible with the homoeopathic principle.

As might be supposed, the allopaths embarked on a production programme in the late 1970s to produce Interferon on a relatively large scale with a view to its administration in macrodoses to boost the body's natural production.

The synthesis of the complex compound being impossible at that time, the original method, in simple terms, employed human blood cells in a thermostatically controlled vessel, which were treated with a disease virus to stimulate them to mimic the natural process of stimulating the production of Interferon in the blood cells. The product was continuously separated and measured in terms of micrograms per litre per hour over a period of up to twenty-four hours.

In 1980, the author approached an allopathic pharmaceutical manufacturing laboratory in order to carry out a research programme using their equipment that would prove not only how homoeopathy works but also that it does work.

The study would involve the addition of a liquid homoeopathic potency added to the system shortly after the addition of the disease virus (in this experiment, an influenza virus, although any virus would suffice). If it could be demonstrated that the addition of the homoeopathic potency increased the rate of formation of Interferon, then the belief that homoeopathic cure was a function of the stimulation of the body's immune system would be strengthened.

Regrettably, at a late stage, the manufacturing laboratories withdrew their co-operation without explanation and the project was abandoned. However, a pilot experiment only was carried out at the University of California, Berkeley, US in 1981 which proved to be positive. The results were never published.

THE NATURE OF CAUSTICUM

A question that has vexed homoeopaths for more than 150 years since it was introduced by Samuel Hahnemann is exactly what is the remedy Causticum.

The efficacy of the remedy itself is not in question and it is widely prescribed and recognized as a minor polycrest. Its action centres on chronic rheumatic conditions and paralysis of single muscles or muscle groups, including the vocal cords, throat, face and bladder. Causticum conditions are characterized by burning, rawness and soreness.

Our observations leave us now in no doubt that the source of the remedy is the impure alkali, potassium hydroxide (caustic potash), with the chemical formula KOH.

Hahnemann titled the remedy Tinctura Acris Sine Kali Causticum. He prepared it by the distillation of a mixture of calcium hydroxide (slaked lime) and potassium bisulphate to produce a viscous, colourless liquid.

The chemical reaction is as follows:

The insoluble white powder of calcium

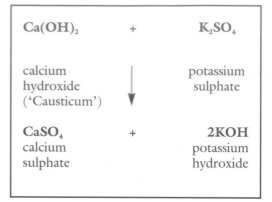

$Ca(OH)_2$ + K_2SO_4

calcium hydroxide ('Causticum') • potassium sulphate

$CaSO_4$ + $2KOH$
calcium sulphate • potassium hydroxide

sulphate forms the residue of the distillation. The tincture of the remedy has the lye smell of potassium hydroxide and its pH value (hydrogen ion concentration) is 11–12 which conforms with a pH of 11 for a 0.1M (0.1 Molar) solution of pure potassium hydroxide, which is strongly alkaline.

Modern laboratory analysis of Causticum tincture showed that neither calcium nor sulphate ions are present, which is consistent with the method of preparation, but a small amount of sodium ions were present. Precise analysis is difficult as potassium hydroxide is deliquescent.

It is certain, therefore, that the remedy Causticum is potassium hydroxide with traces of sodium hydroxide (caustic soda).

HEALING VENOMS

In recent years conventional drug companies have diverted more and more of their research resources from their traditional synthetic approach to a search for natural products. This seems to have resulted from a reluctant recognition that even with all the advances of modern technology nothing can match the diversity and complexity of nature.

Much of this research has been based on the exploration of venoms from a wide variety of spiders, scorpions, snakes, sea creatures and lizards. In keeping with the allopathic approach, however, researchers have exploited these animals for the identification, extraction and isolation of single, specific, poisonous compounds, which may serve as potential drugs when given in large doses. Paradoxically, such natural compounds are generally considered to be only the starting point for the development of new drugs and synthetic derivatives may be modelled for a specific application. Thus, this attention given to natural sources, which might have been seen by homoeopaths as a welcome trend in allopathic drug research, has inevitably drifted back towards the traditional allopathic approach of a single, synthesized substance given in macrodoses.

The homoeopathic ethic demands that its remedies are derived from natural sources and that they represent the whole extract, retaining all the complexity, essence and subtlety of nature that defies the understanding of humankind. Furthermore, only Hahnemannian provings can lead the homoeopath to discover a new remedy and 'clinical provings', except in rare circumstances, are unacceptable. Classical homoeopathy demands that the natural product must be homoeopathically potentized by recognized procedures.

Nevertheless, much of the recent work in this field of drug development could provide clues or the inspiration for the selection of other species of spiders, snakes, scorpions and other creatures as the sources for potential homoeopathic remedies. This approach in no way conflicts with homoeopathic precepts. Without doubt, these venomous creatures could provide a rich source for new homoeopathic remedies.

Existing remedies, many of them great polycrests, are already part of the mainstay of the homoeopathic *Materia Medica*, such as Lachesis mutus (bushmaster snake), Bothrops lanceolatus (yellow viper), Tarantula hispanica, Latrodectus mactans (black widow spider), Latrodectus katipo (California spider), Bufo rana (poison toad), and Scorpion, recently proved by Jeremy Sherr, which is considered to be a very promising new remedy.

A brief review of recent allopathic research in this field might suggest some useful avenues for new homoeopathic remedies with high expectations of successful classical provings.

Spider Remedies

Among the venomous spiders are the most poisonous living creatures on earth and the homoeopathic *Materia Medica* already has some outstanding remedies, including Latrodectus mactans (black widow), Latrodectus hasselti (red back), Aranea diadema (papal cross), Mygale lasiodora (black cuban) and Theridion curassavicum (orange spider). Their keynotes demonstrate a strong action on the nervous system, radiating and chest pain, heart affections and muscular spasms.

Grammostola patulata: The Chilean pink. Tarantula venom, studied by Zeneca, contains complex peptides that inhibit calcium entry into the nerve cells. It is generally accepted that N-type calcium channels control neurotransmitter release and other calcium channels have a fundamental role. The venom could therefore be useful as an analgesic and as a non-addictive alternative to morphine.

Hysterocrates gigas: The large African tarantula, also known as the Cameroon red tarantula, produces a venom which

113

immobilizes its prey. Neurex (US) have focused their work on its use for the treatment of cardio-renal and neurological disorders.

NPS pharmaceuticals have researched components of venom of other spiders. Proteins from these venoms have provided clues for the means to protect brain cells in stroke victims until blood flow to the affected area can be re-established.

Lizard Remedy

Heloderma suspectum: Otherwise known as the Gila monster lizard, Heloderma suspectum injects its venom through hollow fangs. Amylin Pharmaceuticals is developing a synthetic (inevitably!) version of an amino-acid peptide constituent, which stimulates insulin secretion and modulates gastric emptying to slow the entry of ingested sugars into the bloodstream. Its use for treating diabetes and related metabolic disorders is being studied.

Scorpion Remedies

Leuirus quinquestratum: The venom of the giant Israeli scorpion, like all scorpions, has evolved many different toxins, all based on a '37' amino acid peptide called charybdotoxin. This substance is held in shape by three sulphur atom bonds set in its core.

Reasearchers at the University of Alabama have isolated one of these peptides, called chlorotoxin, which blocks chloride ion channels that, if disrupted, cause muscle spasms. It is believed that it could be useful in the treatment of brain cancer.

Contruroides margaritatus: Merck (US) is also studying the constituents of scorpion venoms, notably a peptide called margatoxin which may be of use in the treatment of auto-immune and chronic inflammatory disorders.

Snake Remedies

Homoeopaths are already well served by snake remedies, as we have seen, but we may also consider the following as candidates for provings:

Bothrops jaracusa: The venom of the Brazilian arrowhead viper, an enzyme inhibitor, is a good example of the development of a constituent of a venom by Cushman and Ondetti of the Squibb Corporation for use as an anti-hypertensive agent.

Sistrurus miliarus barbouri: The venom of the south-eastern pygmy rattlesnake has been shown by Schering-Plough to contain a complex heptapeptide protein substance, which has received US Food and Drugs Administration (FDA) approval for use as an anti-coagulation agent in patients suffering from severe cardiovascular diseases, unstable angina and myocardial infarction.

Agkistrodon rhodostoma: BASF Pharmaceuticals isolated a compound, Ancrod, from the venom of this snake, the Malaysian pit viper. It was found that blood did not clot in animals bitten by this snake by removing a protein that augments clot formation from the blood, thus improving blood flow. Blood supply is interrupted to parts of the brain in the course of a stroke and Ancrod may be able to reduce serious neurological damage and reduce the mortality rate.

Agkistrodon contortix: The venom of the southern copperhead viper provides an extracted protein which is currently involved in trials for the treatment of breast cancer by stopping cancer cells adhering to and invading neighbouring cells.

Naja mocambique: Mozambican spitting cobra venom has been studied by the Massachusetts Genetic Institute in the US. A protein isolated from the venom is believed to be of use in developing agents for treating inflammatory disease.

Sea Species Remedies

Conus magnus: The giant carnivorous sea snail has a compound in its venom which is being subjected to trials by Neurex for analgesia and the treatment of strokes.

Physalia physalis: The Portuguese man-of-war jellyfish is an example of a sea anemone whose venom can be up to 75 per cent of the toxicity of cobra venom. Its sting can, in extreme cases, lead to convulsions and death. Recent research has suggested that the venom may be useful in acting on sodium channels in the body.

The Future

Clearly, provings of more animal sources for new homoeopathic remedies should be very fruitful, as the examples mentioned represent only the 'tip of the iceberg'. Furthermore, homoeopathic provings will elicit the whole natural healing power representing the infinite majesty of nature and not simply that of a single synthetic extract. As Kent said, a good poison makes a good medicine!

QUESTIONS

Answers are given on page 187

1. What were the original potencies prescribed by Samuel Hahnemann?

----

2. The old duodecimal system of counting was based on units

of ---

3. The original homoeopathic remedy introduced by Hahnemann

was ---

4. The 'active ingredient' of the remedy in question 3

was ---

5. Name four essential mineral nutrients identified in the twentieth

century:

----

6. The true chemical substance, described as the remedy Calcarea metallicum is in fact

----

7. The remedy Causticum is derived from

----

8. In the crystalline form of the remedy, Graphites, the carbon atoms are arranged in

----

CHAPTER 8
Brief Drug Pictures

The drug picture. Sources of remedies. Origins, polycrests, keynotes, therapeutic durations, constitutions, modalities. Complementary medicines. Antidotes.

THE ESSENTIAL TRIAD OF HOMOEOPATHY

Homoeopathy is a natural therapy with an holistic approach that aims to treat the whole person. To achieve this aim we need to know and understand the whole person.

J. H. Clarke stated that the *Materia Medica* is the *raison d'etre* of the homoeopath and that it is impossible to practice homoeopathy as it should be practised without the aid of a Repertory. The best Repertory is the fullest.

It is not enough to memorize the *Materia Medica* learning proving symptoms by rote. We must consider every remedy in its entirety, not memorize lists of unrelated symptoms. Kent described the study of *Materia Medica* as, at worst, a tedious drudgery. It presents a tremendous challenge to beginners and many new students find it daunting to face the prospect which, of course, is impossible anyway, of learning remedy after remedy from A through to Z.

Every remedy, however, has its own individual character and, as their study progresses, we can build up a drug picture as Dr Margaret Tyler described it, whereby we can begin to understand the true nature of the remedy. We can develop an appreciation of the intrinsic qualities of each natural remedy, its origin, its source, its nuances and foibles. It is for this reason that the procedure for preparing homoeopathic mother tincture requires more than mechanistic scientific rules, important as they are, but also aims to capture the natural substance, whether it be plant, animal or mineral in all its essence and subtleties.

Thus, with experience, every homoeopathic practitioner builds up his or her own picture of each remedy. Simply the mention of the name of a remedy will immediately conjure in the mind a living, exciting individuality of the remedy and the patient to achieve an holistic cure.

I have not, therefore, provided in this chapter a condensed *Materia Medica* since many excellent detailed works are now available (see Bibliography), but instead you will find below a series of drug pictures embracing notes on the origins and source of remedy, and points of special interest, such as underlying miasmic nature. Essential keynotes (which can be learned by the student), duration of therapeutic activity, constitution, complementary remedies and antidotes are also included.

No meaningful study of the *Materia Medicas* can be made without reference to the two other quintessential works, the Organon of Medicine and Repertory. These works form the essential triad of homoeopathy. They are so closely interwoven that no homoeopathic student can aspire to achieve anything worth while without constant cross-referencing between these disciplines (Kishore, 1971).

Although we must first repertorize, the

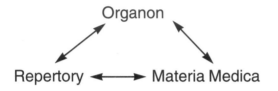

Organon

Repertory ← → Materia Medica

actual prescription is made by reference to the *Materia Medica*. The Repertory is an essential tool only and cannot be considered a substitute for the *Materia Medica*.

THE REMEDIES

The following remedies are listed in alphabetical order:

Abrotanum
Aconitum napellus
Alumina
Apis mellifica
Argentum nitricum
Arnica montana
Arsenicum album
Aurum metallicum
Atropa belladonna
Berberis vulgaris
Bryonia alba
Calcarea carbonica
Calcarea fluorica
Calendula officinalis

Cantharis vesicatoria
Carbo vegetabilis
Caulophyllum
Chamomilla
Chelidonium majus
Cocculus indicus
Conium maculatum
Cuprum metallicum
Drosera rotundfolia
Euphrasia officinalis
Ferrum phosphoricum
Gelsemium sempervirens
Graphites
Hepar sulphuris
Hypericum perforatum
Ignatia amara
Iodum
Ipecacuanha
Kalium bichromicum
Lachesis
Ledum palustre
Lycopodium clavatum
Medorrhinum
Mercurius muriaticum
Natrum muriaticum
Nux vomica
Petroleum
Phosphorus
Psorinum
Pulsatilla nigricans
Rhus toxicodendron
Ruta graveolens
Sepia officinalis
Silicea
Staphysagria
Sulphur
Symphytum officinalis
Taraxacum
Tarantula hispanica
Thuja occidentalis
Tuberculinum
Veratum album
Zincum metallicum

ABROTANUM

Artemisa abrotanum

Common names: Southernwood, Lady's Love
Abbreviation: Abrotanum
Repertory abbreviation: Abrot.

Source/Origin

Evergreen shrub with fragrant foliage and yellow flowers (August to October) found in Europe.

The leaf, stems and young shoots are used to prepare the mother tincture.

Presented in Allen's *Encyclopedia of Materia Medica*, Vol. 1.

Keynotes

Symptoms closely resemble Bryonia and Rhus tox. (qv.). Pleurisy, rheumatic conditions in joints, marasmus of children, lower limb upward, metastasis, diarrhoea (cf. Nat. sulph.). Weakness following influenza.

Epilepsy, gout, haemorrhoids.

Constitution

Not strong constitutionally. Often with children, they are irritable, emaciated, with flabby skin. Anxiety and depression is common. Excitable, loquacious, tending to shout. Sensation as if stomach is hanging or swimming in water.

Modalities

All symptoms < at night. < cold air. < motion

Complementary Remedies

Bryonia, Rhus tox., Scrophularia

Antidotes

None listed.

ACONITE

Aconitum napellus
Common names: Monkshood, Wolfsbane, Helmut Flower
Abbreviation: Acomite
Repertory abbreviation: Acon.

Source/Origin

A great polycrest remedy. Commonly called Monkshood on account of purple flowers resembling a monk's hood.

A perennial herb with perpendicular, tapering roots and upright stem. The purple or dark violet flowers open May to July in temperate climates. The whole flowering plant, including the root, is used in preparing the mother tincture. Contains the very poisonous alkaloid, aconitine. See *Hering's Guiding Symptoms.*

   Proved by Hahnemann.

Keynotes

Acute disease, sudden symptoms. Physical and mental trauma and restlessness. Fright, fear, anxiety. Influenza and sudden colds. Numbness and tingling in limbs and cheeks. Fever, red, hot, swollen skin. Profuse sweating. Great thirst. Hoarse, dry, croup cough. Vertigo with nausea. Headaches, better in open air. Eye infections, tearing, cutting pain.

Therapeutic Duration

Very fast – one hour.

Constitution

A very fearful, anxious apprehensive person with an anxious expression who is very restless, mentally and physically, and worries about minor things. The face may be hot and red. They are prone to colds on exposure to dry, cold weather.

Always fear that some misfortune will happen. The anxiety is inconsolable. Poor memory and becomes confused with his or her thoughts. One cheek pale, other cheek red (cf. Chamomilla).

Modalities

< dry, cold weather < chill < very hot weather < noise.

.< music (e.g. Graphites, Thuja), < warm room < lying on affected side, tobacco smoke, < night (especially midnight).

Complementary Remedies

Arnica, Coffea, Sulphur.

Antidotes

Acidum acet., Belladonna, Berberis, Coffea, Nux vomica, Sulphur.

Note: Aconite is the 'A' of the 'ABC' of children's remedies.

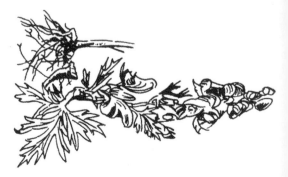

Aconitum napellus

ALUMINA

Common names: Aluminium (aluminum, US) oxide, bauxite
Abbreviation: Alumina
Repertory abbreviation: Alum.

Source/Origin

White, odourless, tasteless, amorphous (without shape) powder. Formula Al_2O_3. Used as a chromatographic matrix. Proved by Hahnemann, Allen's *Encyclopedia of Materia Medica*, Vol. I.

Keynotes

Sluggishness, weariness. Numbness, especially legs (with knees crossed). Constipation (no power to strain – Tyler), hard, knotty stools. Dryness of mucous membranes. Premature ageing. Sore throat in public speaking. Sense of constriction from oesophagus to stomach (Allen) on swallowing food.

Therapeutic Duration

Slow – six weeks to two months.

Constitution

Thin, moody person who may have a red nose and ears. Sluggish in his or her actions with tendency to premature ageing. Eats frequently in small portions. Craves indigestible things such as earth, chalk, clay, rice (Tyler). Easily inebriated with alcohol. Weakly children and girls at puberty (Farrington). Unable to make decisions (Kent).

Modalities

< periodically (e.g. alternate days)
< afternoon and evening.
< potatoes < cold washing > damp weather.

Complementary Remedies

Bryonia, Ferrum met.

Antidotes

Bryonia, Camphor, Chamomilla, Ipecacuanha.

APIS MELLIFICA

Common name: Honey bee
Abbreviation: Apis mel
Repertory abbreviation: Apis

Source/Origin

Whole, live worker honey bee (with sting) immersed in alcohol/water solution. The bee is not compressed. Bees preferably selected when active. Rare example of a live insect being used in the preparation of a remedy. Hering recommended using the sting alone. Introduced in Allen's Encyclopedia, Vol.1 and Elements of a New *Materia Medica*, p.442 (Marcy).

Keynotes

All symptoms characteristic of the sting of the bee. Pains like bee stings with thirst and burning (Guernsey). Redness and swelling with stinging and burning pain (Hering). Sharp, stinging pains act on entire skin of the body and mucous membranes (Kent). Great throat medicine. Violent cases of diptheria with oedematous swelling (Nash). Vertigo. Headache (Allen). Wasp stings. Right-sided remedy.

Therapeutic Duration

Fast.

Constitution

Weak constitutionally. Active women, children and young girls with sensitive skin. Awkward people but careful. May be indifferent, jealous (cf. Lachesis) or suspicious.

Modalities

> open air > cold bathing > removing clothes, > walking > sitting erect.

 < heat. < pressure < touch < after sleep < heated rooms < hot bath < getting wet < right side.

Complementary Remedies

Natrum mur.

Antidotes

Cantharis, Ipecacuanha, Lachesis, Ledum, Natrum mur., Plantago, Acid Lac.

ARGENTUM NITRICUM

Common name: Silver nitrate
Abbreviation: Argent nit.
Repertory abbreviation: Arg-n

Source/Origin

Colourless crystals of silver nitrate; chemical formula, $AgNO_3$. Odourless, bitter-tasting, tending to turn brown in daylight (keep in amber glass container). Very soluble in water and soluble in alcohol. The colourless mother tincture is prepared by dissolving the crystals in water.

Keynotes

Trembling (in affected parts). Flatulence with abdominal distention and belching (explosive) (cf. Carbo veg.). Neurosis. Claustrophobia. Premature aged look. Anaemia. Nervous anticipation ('Funk Remedy') (Tyler).

Therapeutic Duration

Medium – one month.

Constitution

A prematurely aged person with withered, drawn, dry skin and possibly blotches. Nervous, irrational and impulsive, always wanting to do things in a hurry. Fears forthcoming events, particularly public appearances and apprehensive of disease or failure. They have a great liking for sweets (candies) and salty foods. Cannot stand heat. Feel that death is always near (Kent) (cf. Aconite).

Modalities

< lying on right side < before events < warmth < at night.
< cold food < sweets (candies) < during periods.
< emotions < (cf. Gelsemium) < left side < rising from sitting.
> fresh air > cold > pressure > standing or walking.

Complementary Remedies

None listed.

Antidotes

Arsen alb., Calc. carb., Lycopodium, Natrum mur., Merc. sol., Phosphorus, Pulsatilla, Rhus tox., Sepia, Silica, Sulphur.

ARNICA MONTANA

Common names: Mountain arnica, Leopardsbane, Fallkraut
Abbreviation: Arnica
Repertory abbreviation: Arn.

Source/Origin

A small perennial herb with tubular yellow florets with a pleasant, sweet, aromatic odour, growing only on higher ground on hills or lower mountain slopes. Hahnemann picked the plant in the foothills of the Erz mountains and pressed it in a book. The fresh, whole plant is used to prepare the mother tincture. Sometimes called the *Sportsman's Remedy*.

Keynotes

Physical trauma. Traumatic injuries. Bruises applied topically (when skin is not broken). Contusions. Strains and sprains. Muscular wear and tear. Exhaustion after strenuous exertion. Soreness. Lameness. Wasp stings (Tyler)(cf. Apis).
Some evidence of causing hair growth on limbs (Ussher).

Therapeutic Duration

Fast – about one week.

Constitution

Weak constitutionally. Athletic type of person who over-exerts himself or herself and feels body is beaten. The Arnica person always finds his or her bed too hard even if it is soft. Liable to travel sickness.

Modalities

< least touch < motion < rest < wine < damp < cold.
> lying down > rest > lying with head low.
< night.

Complementary Remedies

Aconite, Ipecacuanha, Veratrum alb., Hypericum, Rhus tox.

Antidotes

Aconite, Arsen alb., Camphor, Cinchona, Ignatia, Ipecacuanha.

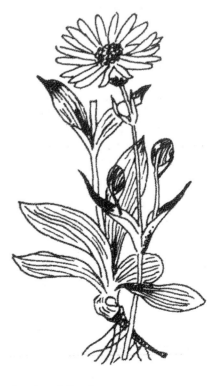

Arnica Montana

124

ARSENICUM ALBUM

Common name: Arsenous acid anhydride
Abbreviation: Arsenic trioxide
Repertory abbreviation: Ars.

Source/Origin

White or transparent, amorphous crystalline powder. Formula As_2O_3. Very poisonous.

Originally proved by Hahnemann, Allen's *Encyclopedia of Materia Medica*, Vol. 2.

A major polycrest remedy. Not to be prescribed at potencies less than 3X.

Keynotes

Deep acting on every organ and tissue. Restlessness. Exhaustion (even after slight exertion), low vitality. Burning pain – eyes, throat, stomach, rectum. Asthma, fear, fright, anguish. Skin affections – psoriasis – dry, rough, scaly eruptions. Night aggravation.

Therapeutic Duration

Slow – two to three months.

Constitution

Temperamentally like a thoroughbred race-horse, nervous, highly strung, perspiring easily and capable of tremendous bursts of activity for short periods (Coulter). Neat, clean orderly person with precise movements, piercing eyes, aquiline nose, delicate pale skin, fine boned, fine haired, balding. He or she is elegant with fine taste in clothes, wine, manners, but fastidious and very tidy (folds clothes after use). Obsessive cleanliness. Perfectionist in himself or herself and demanding same of others. Authoritarian and immoderate. Anxious, often miserable hypochondriac who fears death. Always wants to talk about their health and will constantly seek treatment from several practitioners. Even can *enjoy* poor health! Groundless fears about everything. Workaholic business person (cf. Nux vom.). Competitive. Very organized and sensitive to environment.

Loyal, very intelligent, domineering and intolerant. Sips drinks (cf. Sulphur). Archetype: Samuel Hahnemann.

Modalities

< lying on affected side < light < ascending stairs < midnight to 3am < wet weather < after midnight < cold < cold drinks < seashore < right side > heat > head elevated > warm drinks > lying with head high.

Complementary Remedies

Rhus tox., Carbo veg., Phosphorus, Thuja, Secale.

Antidotes

Sulphur, Cinchona, Euphrasia, Graphites, Ferrum met., Iodum, Hepar sulph., Merc. sol., Nux vom., Tabacum, Veratrum alb., Opium.

AURUM METALLICUM

Common name: Gold metal
Abbreviation: Aurum met.
Repertory abbreviation: Aur.

Source/Origin

Bright yellow metal which is malleable and ductile. Dissolves in aqua regia. Triturated in powder form up to 7X potency, then converted to liquid 8X potency in alcohol water. Before the advent of homoeopathy gold was used as an anti-venereal remedy, particularly for syphilis.

Keynotes

Severe depression with thoughts of suicide. Heart affections, palpitation. Arteriosclerosis. Hypertension. Rapid irregular pulse. Photophobia. Nasal problems. Violent headaches. Swelling of testicles.

General features relate to the mind and such as to relate to the tissues of the body in general (Kent).

Therapeutic Duration

Slow – up to two months.

Constitution

Intelligent, intellectual person, good in business affairs who broods privately on his or her problems and cannot communicate them. Deep depressions bordering on insanity or suicide caused by anxiety, trauma, latent syphilis or failure of business or relationship and loss of property. Takes a pessimistic view of everything. Mood swings, peevish–cheerful, happy–sad. (cf. lithium carb.)

Modalities

< night (headache) < cold weather < winter. > open air (cf. Pulsatilla) > becoming warm > cold washing.

Complementary Remedies

Aurum salts, e.g. Aurum mur.

Antidotes

Belladonna, China, Cuprum met., Acid nitricum, Phosphorus Spigelia, Pulsatilla, Cocculus.

BELLADONNA

Atropa belladonna

Common name: Deadly nightshade
Abbreviation: Belladonna
Repertory abbreviation: Bell.

Source/Origin

A major polycrest remedy. Large perennial herb with thick fleshy root. Bell-shaped flowers and black, shiny berries. The berries contain the very poisonous alkaloid, Atropine (hence Atropa). One berry can kill a child and three berries can kill a horse.

Belladonna *'Beautiful Lady'* so named from the habit of women in Renaissance Italy who used the juice of the berries on their eyelids as a cosmetic.

The first 'proving' concerned King Macbeth of Scotland. After the invasion by Danes in the year 1100 he called a truce in the battle and sent wine to the enemy as a sign of goodwill. In the morning the invaders suffered delirium, headaches, bulging eyes, redness of face, etc. and were promptly defeated. Their wine had been laced with the juice of Belladonna!

Keynotes

Primary action on mind and head. Acute conditions of sudden onset. Heat, redness, swelling. Fever. Throbbing and burning pains. Stabbing, *throbbing* headaches. Affects entire nervous system. Inflammation of brain, liver, intestines with violent heat. Vertigo. Moving rheumatic pain. Scarlet fever. Sensitivity to all impressions – light, noise, jar, touch, temperature, damp.

Therapeutic Duration

Very fast – one day to one week.

Constitution

Active, intellectual people. Ruddy face and neck, with staring eyes. Children. Very sensitive. Symptoms are generally worse on the right side (e.g. headache in right temple).

Modalities

< before storms < left side < motion < light < jarring (even the bed) < motion of eyes < after 3pm < bending forward < lying down < swallowing < talking
> keeping head high.

Complementary Remedies

Calcarea carbonica, Hepar sulph., Variolinum.

Antidotes

Aconite, Coffea, Hyoscymas, Merc. sol., Pulsatilla, Sabadilla

NOTE: Belladonna is the 'B' of the 'ABC' of children's remedies. (A=Aconite, C=Chamomilla).

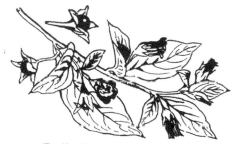

Atropa Belladonna

BERBERIS VULGARIS

Common names: Barberry, pepperidge bush
Abbreviation: Berberis
Repertory abbreviation: Berb.

Source/Origin

A deciduous, spiny shrub indigenous to Europe, Asia and north-east North America, with grey, upright branches and pale yellow roots. The drooping flowers are bright yellow with red glands and the fruits are oblong, scarlet and sour. Kidney-shaped berries. The mother tincture is prepared from the fruit and roots.

Keynotes

Kidney affections, radiating, stitching pain with bubbling sensation in kidney region, worse for pressure (cf. Solidago). Kidney stones. Liver affections. Bladder affections. Gallstones. Smooth warts. Eczema on hands. Lumbago. Shifting, variable pain in all parts. Fits into the gouty, rheumatic sphere (Kent). Sensation – *as if* a tight cap pressing on entire scalp.

Therapeutic Duration

Medium – up to one month.

Constitution

People of sickly appearance with sunken cheeks and grey or bluish colour around the eyes (Gibson). Apathetic, listless and lethargic, they easily become fatigued with mental effort and have a poor memory. Bad tempered, disliking too much conversation, they are inclined to cry. They are nervous, particularly at dusk, and easily become frightened.

Modalities

< motion < sitting < jars < driving cars < night < pressure < fatigue < standing > open air.

Complementary Remedies

None listed.

Antidotes

Camphor, Belladonna.

BRYONIA

Bryonia alba/Bryonia dioica

Common names: White bryony, wild bryony, wild hops
Abbreviation: Bryonia
Repertory abbreviation: Bry.

Source/Origin

A perennial climbing vine with a branched root, alternating leaves and small greenish-yellow flowers developing round, black berries. Indigenous to central and southern Europe.

The mother tincture is prepared from the powdered root collected before flowering. The sub-species alba and dioica are considered to be identical therapeutically. A polycrest remedy.

Keynotes

Stitching and tearing pain. All mucous membranes are dry (e.g. parched lips and mouth). Bursting headache (*'as if hit by a hammer'*). Stomach sensitive to touch (*'as if there is a stone'*). Dyspepsia. Dry, hacking cough. Bronchitis. Stiff, painful swollen joints. Rheumatic pain. Nose bleeds (morning and during periods).

Therapeutic Duration

Medium – one to three weeks.

Constitution

The Bryonia type is an irritable, humourless person, easily angered, with a dark complexion and hair. Often displays a movement of the mouth as if chewing and has dry, cracked lips. He or she over-eats rich foods, wanting foods that are not available and has digestive problems. Children generally do not wish to be carried.

Modalities

< warmth < morning < exertion < touch < hot weather < eating and drinking < motion.
> lying on painful side > pressure > cold > rest.

Complementary Remedies

Alumina, Rhus tox.

Antidotes

Acidum mur., Aconite, Camphor, Chamomilla, Chelidonium, Clematis, Coffea, Ignatia, Nux vom., Pulsatilla, Rhus tox., Senega.

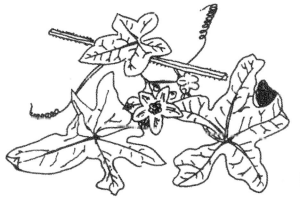

Bryonia alba

CALCAREA CARBONICA

Calcarea carbonica ostrearum

Common name: Calcium carbonate
Abbreviation: Calc. carb.
Repertory abbreviation: Calc.

Source/Origin

Impure calcium carbonate taken from the soft middle layer of the oyster shell, washed with pure water and dried.

Chemical symbol, $CaCO_3$. Fine white, odourless powder.

The remedy was prepared and proved by Hahnemann. Allen's Encyclopedia, Vol. II. Potencies are prepared by trituration.

Keynotes

Mental or physical exhaustion. Nutritional problems. Obesity. Corpulence.

Bulimia. Swollen tonsils with sour taste. Skin affections. Relapses or impaired convalescence. Thyroid conditions. Constipation. Loss of sense of smell.

Therapeutic Duration

Slow – up to two months.

Constitution

Constitutional remedy 'par excellence' (Boericke).

The Calcarea type is fat, fair haired, flabby with pale, chalky skin. He/she perspires easily. Weeps easily over trifles. The handshake is cold, moist and clammy (like the inside of the oyster). Prone to cramps and muscular spasms. Forgetful, apprehensive, anxious and obstinate. Averse to work but once getting started acquits him or herself well. Slightest mental effort causes headache and hot head. Very sensitive to cold.

Dislikes leaving home. Children crave eggs and indigestible substances – chalk, soil etc. (cf. Alumina). Dislikes meat – possibly vegetarian.

Modalities

< exertion < mental or physical effort < ascending stairs < cold < water < washing < moist air < morning < after eating.
> closing eyes > dry > lying on painful side > darkness.

Complementary Remedies

Belladonna, Rhus tox., Lycopodium, Silica.

Antidotes

Acidum nit., Bryonia, Camphor, Cinchona, Ipecacuanha, Nux vom., Sepia, Sulphur.

CANNABIS INDICA

Indian hemp, Marijuanha, Cannabis

Source/Origin

The Ismali sect, known as 'The Assassins' used the drug in the eleventh and twelfth centuries to stimulate them to ruthlessly kill their enemies. The Zulus used it to inspire their Impi warriors to massacre whole communities, including the British Army at Isandlwanha in 1879.

A strong growing plant, growing throughout the world, but particulary in Iran, Malaysia and South America. Large palmate leaves with five serrated leaflets and small, greenish flowers. The other tincture is prepared from the flowering tops of the plant. This hallucinatory drug has a strong affinity for the nervous system. Its effects range from intense exaltation to peaceful contemplation or uncontrollable agitation.

Keynotes

Vertigo with disturbed vision.
Extreme drowsiness.
Deep, throbbing headache (cf. Belladonna).
Tinnitis with buzzing, ringing or throbbing.
Salivation – thick, white, frothy and sticky.
Dark, painful periods with backache.
Increased libido.
Variable pulse.
Paralysis of lower extremities (cf.Conium).
Sensation – *skin on face feels tightly drawn or stretched across the bones.*

Therapeutic Duration

Fast – up to one week.

Constitution

A weary, exhausted appearance with drowsiness and a desire to lie down or walking with a stoop. The pupils are dilated with a fixed stare and redness in the eyes.
Cannabis types may shake their heads involuntarily and lose the thread of their conversation (cf. Natrum mur.) with absent-mindedness. Extremely loquacious (cf. Lachesis), with uncontrollable laughter.
Ecstacy alternates with depression.
Cannot bear heat and is liable to profuse perspiration.
NOTE: *May grind teeth during sleep.*

Modalities

< heat < dark < noise < coffee < alcohol < tobacco smoke < morning < lying on right side < urinating.
> walking outdoors (mental) > lying down > freah air > cold water > rest.

Complementary Remedies

None recorded.

Antidotes

Camphor merc, sol.

CALCAREA FLUORICA

Common name: Calcium fluoride
Abbreviation: Calc. fluor.
Repertory abbreviation: Calc-f

Source/Origin

Soluble, white powder occurs naturally as fluorospar – chemical formula CaF_2 – compound of calcium and fluorine, both essential nutrients. Now recognized as an agent for reducing dental decay. Important tissue remedy. A constituent on the surface of bones. The mother tincture is prepared by trituration up to potency of 7X.

Keynotes

Induration, threatening suppuration. Varicose veins. Bone malnutrition. Toothache. Acute indigestion. Croupy cough. Chronic lumbago. Hodgkin's disease. Bleeding piles.

Therapeutic Duration

Constitution

No strong constitutional features. Men or women, dark or fair. Depression, anxiety, particularly in fear of financial ruin and poverty. Indecisive. May have poor teeth.

Modalities

> heat > gentle movement > warm drinks > rubbing.
< closing eyes.
< rest < damp weather < changes in weather < cold drinks.

Complementary Remedies

Conium, Rhus tox.

CALENDULA OFFICINALIS

Common name: Marigold (common or garden)
Abbreviation: Calendula
Repertory abbreviatio: Calen.

Source/Origin

Whole flowering plant of common or garden marigold. In France the plant is cut just above the ground. Annual flowering plant with oblong leaves and yellow to deep orange flowers, closing at night. The plant has a high moisture content producing much succus on maceration. Recognized as a great healer for surface wounds for more than two hundred years.

Keynotes

Lacerated wounds. Rapid healing of skin cuts, sores and abrasions by topical application as calendula cream (potency 1X or 2X). Sterilizer for wounds. Reduces local pain. First degree burns and scalds.

Therapeutic Duration

Constitution

Weak constitutionally. Kent wrote 'there are no constitutional symptoms to prescribe on and a proving is nearly worthless'. Depressed, easily frightened, irritable people who dislike cold damp weather. Hands are cold.

NOTE. Calendula mother tincture with an equal volume of Hypericum mother tincture (called Hypercal) is an excellent healant.

Modalities

< damp weather < cloudy weather < bending neck to one side.

Complementary Remedies

Hepar Sulphuris.

Antidotes

Arnica.

CANTHARIS VESICATORIA

Common names: Spanish fly, blister beetle
Abbreviation: Cantharis
Repertory abbreviation: Canth.

Source/Origin

Introduced by Hahnemann. Allen's *Encyclopedia Materia Medica*, Vol. II. A golden yellow-green insect about half-an-inch long whose habitat is mainly Spain, Southern Europe and South West Asia. The mother tincture is prepared from the dried powdered insect. Regarded as an aphrodisiac by many lay people.

Keynotes

Prime action on urinary and sexual organs. Inflammations associated with bladder irritation. Fiery, staring look in eyes, burning pain (throat, vagina), short, hacking cough, burning in urination, nymphomania, cystitis, burns and scalds. Kidney affections.

Therapeutic Duration

Medium – one month.

Constitution

Sensitive persons with a pale or yellowish complexion and a staring look (cf. Lachesis) and death-like appearance. Anxiety with irritability and restlessness. Always attempts to start doing something but usually fails. Fiery sexual desire and anger with paroxysms of rage and extravagant gestures.

Modalities

< touch < urinating < coffee.
> rubbing > sexual intercourse.

Complementary Remedies

Camphor.

Antidotes

Aconite, Apis met., Pulsatilla.

CARBO VEGETABILIS

Common name :Vegetable charcoal
Abbreviation: Carbo veg.
Repertory abbreviation: Carb-v

Source/Origin

Black porous carbon with woody appearance prepared by burning birch or beech wood under controlled conditions and washing and drying. Triturated up to 7X potency, then potentized in liquid form. Contains traces of mineral salts.

Proved originally by Hahnemann. Sometimes described as the 'Corpse Reviver' (Tyler).

Keynotes

Deep-acting, long-acting antipsoric remedy (Kent).

Asthma. Burning pain in veins, capilliaries, head, cold knees, nose and ears cold, and offensive breath. Haemorrhoids. Complete collapse – skin cold and blue – even in extremes. Flatulence (more than any other remedy!), with putrid smell and feeling of obstruction. Distended abdomen. Hoarseness.

Never really recovered from a previous illness.

Therapeutic Duration

Slow – up to two months.

Constitution

Sluggish, fat, lazy person, liable to suffer from varicose veins. Poor circulation also causes bluish, cold skin. Old people in states of collapse. Slow digestion with tendency to flatulence and belching and very distended abdomen.

Modalities

> cold > open windows < warm, damp weather < fatty foods < open air < singing < 4 to 5pm < brandy < morning.

Complementary Remedies

Drosera, Kali carb., Phosphorus.

Antidotes

Arsen alb., Coffea, Lachesis, Camphor, Ferrum met.

CAULOPHYLLUM

Common names: Blue cohosh, squaw root
Abbreviation: Caulophyllum
Repertory abbreviation: Caul.

Source/Origin

The mother tincture is prepared from the root of the plant. Closely related to Actea racemosa (black cohosh).

Keynotes

Uterine spasms (cf. Secale – *Ergot*). Rheumatic condition in small joints and muscles. Thrush, locally and internally. Stomach pains and dyspepsia.
Speeds progress of labour. Profuse periods, late or early. Pains in inguinal region.
See Chapter 6, Case 9.

Constitution

Women's remedy, with particular affinity for pregnant women.

Liable to abort in early months of pregnancy. Weak contractions of the uterus ('too feeble to extract the contents', Kent). She is sensitive to cold and likes warm clothing (contrast with Pulsatilla). Suffers from cold feet. Tends to become hysterical, excitable, fretful, nervous and apprehensive. Small joints prone to rheumatism, stiffness and swelling.

Modalities

< night < stooping < coffee.

CHAMOMILLA

Common names: Bitter chamomile, German chamomile, Wild chamomile.
Abbreviation: Chamomilla
Repertory abbreviation: Cham.

Source/Origin

Annual herb with white strap-shaped flowers with an aromatic odour flowering in September. Member of the daisy family, fast growing with seed produced in a few months. There is an affinity for the nervous system. The whole dried plant is used for the preparation of the mother tincture.

SOURCE: Hahnemann's *Materia Medica* Pura.

Keynotes

Hypersensitivity. Irritability. Earache. Teething infants (one cheek red and hot, the other pale and cold (cf. Aconite, Calc. phos.). Thirst. Biliousness. Colic. Dry, tickling cough

Therapeutic Duration

Medium – up to one month.

Constitution

Sensitive people easily offended or excited – sudden, spiteful irritability (Guernsey). Impatient people with exaggerated response to stimulation and poor appetite common. May sleep with eyes wide open. The Chamomilla child 'doubles up, kicks and screams, wants this, wants that and throws away toys' (Hahnemann).

Modalities

< coffee (Kent) < warm drinks < fluids < heat < anger < open air < night.
> being nursed or carried > warm wet weather.

Complementary Remedies

Belladonna.

Antidotes

Aconite, Alum, Borax, Cinchona, Cocculus, Coffea, Colocynthis, Conium, Ignatia, Pulsatilla, Valerian.

NOTE: Chamomilla is the 'C' of the ABC of children's remedies. See Aconite and Belladonna.

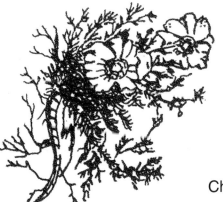

Chamomilla

COCCULUS INDICUS

Common names: Indian cockle, Indian berry
Abbreviation: Cocculus
Repertory abbreviation: Cocc.

Source/Origin

A woody, climbing plant with small, greenish-yellow flowers and large leaves indigenous to East Indies and Malaya. Sweet scented. The seeds and fruit are used to prepare the mother tincture. Contains poisonous alkaloids *menispermine* and *paramenispermine*. Used to 'spike drinks in low dives in days gone by' or to stupefy fish by throwing the fruit into the water (Gibson).

Keynotes

Prostration with 'all-gone' sensation often induced by lack of sleep. Vertigo with nausea << motion. Profuse leucorrhoea. Back pain (small of back) and pain in shoulders and arms. Painful contracture of limbs. Travel sickness (see below).

Therapeutic Duration

Medium – one month.

Constitution

Fair-haired females, sensitive and romantic teenagers (cf. Pulsatilla). Problems during pregnancy, with nausea and backache common. All symptoms are worse for travel, particularly by sea, but also in cars.

Modalities

< eating < loss of sleep < open air < smoking < swimming < touch, noise. < jar (cf Bell) < afternoon.
< during menstruation < travel (cars, ships) < emotional upset.
> lying down > silence.

Complementary Remedies

Pulsatilla, Ignatia.

Antidotes

Coffea, Nux vomica, Cuprum met., Chamomilla, Causticum, Camphor.

CONIUM MACULATUM

Common name: Poison hemlock
Abbreviation: Conium
Repertory abbreviation: Con.

Source/Origin

Proved by Hahnemann in 1825. Conium maculatum (mottled or spotted) is a large, branching herb with white flowers. Resembles parsley, hence sometimes called 'poison parsley' and many deaths reported by people who have mistakenly eaten it.

The constituent alkaloid *coniine* is very poisonous. The first 'proving' concerned the philosopher Socrates who was executed by being given a chalice of the extract of hemlock. It was recorded by Plato who described the resulting paralysis moving upwards, leading ultimately to death by asphyxiation through paralysis of the respiratory muscles.

Keynotes

Trembling, palpitations, loss of strength, stiffness of legs, ascending paralysis, senility, vertigo (on lying down), photophobia, effects of celibacy.

Therapeutic Duration

Slow – one to two months.

Constitution

Older people, particularly those leading celibate lives. Widowers and widows. No interest in work or play. Nervous conditions are common. Weakness of limbs with muscular weakness and drooping gait. Likes to sit with feet up. Liable to suffer menstrual and menopausal problems.

Modalities

< lying down > turning < celibacy < menses < mental exertion
> in the dark > pressure > motion.

Complementary Remedies

Baryta carb., Hydrastis, Kali phos.

Antidotes

Acid nit., Coffea, Dulcamara.

CUPRUM METALLICUM

Common name: Copper metal
Abbreviation: Cuprum
Repertory abbreviation: Cupr.

Source/Origin

Reddish-brown, lustrous metal that is malleable and ductile. Symbol Cu. Name derived from Cyprus. Coated with green basic copper carbonate on exposure to air. Alloyed with zinc for brass. Originally proved by Hahnemann, Allen's Encyclopedia, Vol. 4 and The Chronic Diseases, 3rd edn. Lower potencies up to 6X prepared by trituration.

Keynotes

Nausea. Cramps, especially calf muscles. Spasmodic conditions, for example spasmodic asthma, muscular spasms, paralysis. Convulsions followed by extreme mental and physical exhaustion. Dry cough with violent thirst and thick and sticky saliva. Angina pectoris.

Therapeutic Duration

Slow – six to seven weeks.

Constitution

People with reddish faces and liable to jerking in limbs. Hips and limbs may have a bluish tinge. They may have speech difficulties with stammering and are slow to reply to a question. Easily lose their temper and moods vary widely between sullen, loquacious and malicious. Children are typically spoilt, changeable moods, dissatisfied and disorderly. Chilly people who may twitch and jerk in their sleep.

Modalities

< cold air < cold winds < touch < evening < night.
< before periods < vomiting < contact.
> perspiring > cold water.

Complementary Remedies

Calc. carb.

Antidotes

Belladonna, Camphor, Cicuta, Cinchona, Cocculus, Veratrum alb., Conium, Dulcamara, Ipecacuanha, Merc. sol., Nux vomica, Pulsatilla.

DROSERA ROTUNDIFOLIA

Common name: Sundew
Abbreviation: Drosera
Repertory abbreviation: Dros.

Source/Origin

An insectivorous herb with tufted basal leaves covered in glandular, sensitive hairs, which secrete a fluid to entrap insects. Proved by Hahnemann in 1805, he described the remedy as one of the most powerful medicinal herbs in our zone. The whole plant is used.

Sheep prove the remedy with the acquisition of a violent cough when grazing in pastures where the plant abounds (Tyler).

Keynotes

Whooping cough (spasmodic cough) – main remedy. Laryngitis, Pain in hip joints, tubercular glands, bones and joints, constipation, muscular and limb pain, restlessness, chronic asthma, scar tissue (cf. Graphites and Silicea), exhaustion, cramps.

Therapeutic Duration

Medium – up to one month.

Constitution

Quiet, reserved person with an uneasy, mistrustful disposition. Anxious, as if persecuted, and when he or she is alone. Always seeks company. Shivers easily, particularly at rest. Feels the bed is hard (cf. Arnica, Pyrogen). Easily angered, even under the slightest provocation.

Modalities

< 7 to 8pm < after midnight < lying down < drinking.
< laughing < warmth.

Complementary Remedies

Nux vomica.

Antidotes

Camphor.

141

EUPHRASIA OFFICINALIS

Common name: Eyebright
Abbreviation: Euphrasia
Repertory abbreviation: Euphr.

Source/Origin

An annual plant with purple or white flowers indigenous to Newfoundland. The name Euphrasia is derived from the Greek word 'cheerfulness'. Recognized as an eye remedy since ancient times, hence 'eyebright'.

The mother tincture is prepared from the whole plant.

Keynotes

Eye affections – conjunctivitis, lachrymation, coryza, cataract, inflammation, swelling of lower lid. Granular eyelids as if dust in the eyes. Acute catarrh, sneezing. Intense, throbbing headaches. Constipation. Measles (first stages).

Painful periods. Prostate (frequent urination at night).

Therapeutic Duration

Fast – up to one week.

Constitution

Weak constitutionally. Indolent, taciturn people who dislike talking and avoid bright lights. Hypochondriacs who easily become depressed. Prone to eye problems and drowsiness and yawning during the daytime. Always chilly and cannot get warm in bed (Kent).

Modalities

< lying down < during night < after sleep < touch < evening (coryza) < indoors < warmth < light.
> at night (cough) > in bed > getting out of bed > open air (except coryza) > coffee > darkness.

Complementary Remedies

None recorded.

Antidotes

Camphor, Pulsatilla, Causticum.

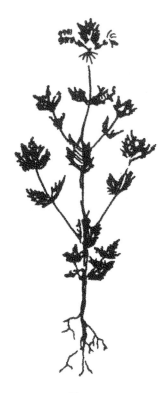

Euphrasia officinalis

FERRUM PHOSPHORICUM

Common name: Ferric phosphate
Abbreviation: Ferrum phos.
Repertory abbreviation: Ferr-p

Source/Origin

White, greyish-white, light pink or greenish-blue orthorhomhic or monoclinic crystals or powder. Ferric phosphate, formula $Fe_3(PO_4)$. $8H_2O$ occurs naturally with ferrous phosphate and hydrated iron oxides.

Introduced by Dr Schüssler and proved by Dr Moffat, *Allen's Encyclopedia*, Vol. X.

Keynotes

Dull, hammering headache. Bronchitis and catarrhal affections. Hoarseness, Laryngitis. All inflammations (first stages). Poor appetite. Diarrhoea. Enuresis.

Therapeutic Duration

Slow – one to two months.

Constitution

Nervous, sensitive, anaemic people of slim build or emaciated with flushing, florid faces.

Easily take cold and prone to respiratory affections, especially bronchitis in young children. Talkative persons with good humour, but liable to get over-excited. Mood changes swiftly from pleasant to quarrelling. Slow mentally with difficulty in remembering names, etc. Capricious appetite with aversion to certain foods is common, including meat, cakes, tea and milk.

Modalities

< cough < eating < night < 4 to 6am < touch < jar (cf. Belladonna) < motion < right side > cold applications > cold drinks > gentle motion > lying down.

Complementary Remedies

Cinchona.

Antidotes

Arsen alb., Sulphur.

GELSEMIUM SEMPERVIRENS

Common name: Yellow yasmine
Abbreviation: Gelsemium
Repertory abbreviation: Gels.

Source/Origin

Important polycrest remedy. Evergreen vine growing up to 8m (24ft) high. Bright yellow flowers that are very fragrant. Forms a fruit, then flat, winged seeds. The rhizome is used to prepare the mother tincture. Indigenous to North America. Introduced to homoeopathy by Henry in 1852 and proved by Douglas a year later.

Keynotes

Action on the entire nervous system. Motor paralysis. Muscular weakness. Nervous headache. Influenza-like symptoms (also as a prophylactic against flu). Measles. Trembling in all limbs. Insomnia.

Therapeutic Duration

Medium – one month.

Constitution

Languid, sluggish people with drooping eyelids and poor eyesight. Easily fatigued with trembling. Especially active for children and young people. Nervous apprehension (cf. Argent nit.).

NOTE: Gelsemium colds develop several days after exposure, whereas the Aconite cold comes on after a few hours (Kent).

Modalities

< damp weather < before storms < emotion < excitement < bad news < 10am.
> bending forward > profuse urination > open air.
> stimulants > continued motion.

Complementary Remedies

Ignatia.

Antidotes

Cinchona, Coffea, Digitalis.

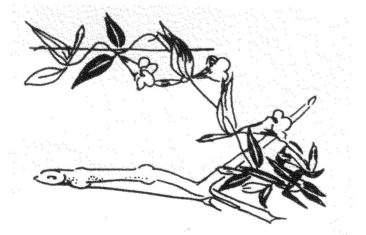

Gelsemium
sempervirens

GRAPHITES

Common names: Graphite, plumbago, black lead
Abbreviation: Graphites
Repertory abbreviation: Graph.

Source/Origin

Allotropic form of the pure mineral non-metallic element carbon. Symbol C. Blackish, grey powder. Hahnemann stated he used the *'pure lead of an English pencil'* as his source. Mother tincture prepared in solid form by trituration. See diagrams, Chapter 8. Powerful antipsoric remedy.

Keynotes

Eczema. Oozing eruptions with sticky exudation (particularly behind ears and earlobes). Psoriasis. Every injury suppurates. Wheezing. Bronchitic patients. Swollen, red eyelids. Strange, rare and peculiar sensation: *'As if there is a cobweb on my face'.*

Therapeutic Duration

Constitution

Especially for overweight flabby people, anaemic with redness of face with fair complexion and a tendency to skin affections. Timid people affected by music that makes them weep. Prefers cold drinks with digestive problems and flatulence. Aversion to meat and sweets may nauseate. Likes to loosen clothing. Females prone to sore, cracked nipples. Fingernails an important indicator – brittle, thick, rough, cracked, deformed with black marks. Children take colds easily.

The Graphites child patient fidgets then wanders round the consulting room, grabbing everything in sight, bringing things to the floor, showing impudence to his mother's reprimands (Hahnemann)

Modalities

< warmth < at night < during and after menstruation < music < lying down > in the dark > wrapping up > eating.

Complementary Remedies

Arsen alb., Causticum, Ferrum met., Hepar sulph., Lycopodium.

Antidotes

Aconite, Nux vomica, Arsen alb., Cinchona.

HEPAR SULPHURIS

Common name: Calcium sulphide
Abbreviation: Hepar sulph.
Repertory abbreviation: Hep.

Source/Origin

Otherwise known as Hahnemann's calcium sulphide or Hepar sulphuris calcareum. White, porous, amorphous (without shape) powder of calcium sulphide, chemical formula CaS. Prepared and introduced by Hahnemann, Allen's Encyclopedia, Vol. IV. Prepared from powdered oyster shells (Calcium carbonate) and sulphur at white heat. Potencies are prepared by trituration.

Keynotes

Tendency to suppuration with all injuries. Abcesses. Offensive discharges. Cold sores. Sensitive to all external impressions. Very chilly. Mucous membranes. Eruptions and glandular swellings.

Therapeutic Duration

Slow – forty to fifty days.

Constitution

Fast talkers who are easily irritated. Males and females with blond hair and unhealthy skin. Always feel chilly and respond to the slightest draught or cool air, even to imagine a cold wind was blowing on some part of their body. 'The slightest thing put him into a violent passion and he could have murdered someone without hesitation' (Hahnemann).

NOTE: Hepar sulph. closely resembles Silicea.

Modalities

< dry cold winds < cool air < slightest draught < touch < lying on painful side.
> damp weather > wrapping up > warmth > after food.

Complementary Remedies

Calendula.

Antidotes

Belladonna, Chamomilla, Silicea, Acetic acid, Citric acid.

HYPERICUM PERFORATUM

Common name: St John's wort
Abbreviation: Hypericum
Repertory abbreviation: Hypcr.

Source/Origin

Proved by Dr Muller and introduced into homoeopathic practice in 1837. In the Middle Ages bunches of Hypericum were hung over the front door of houses or strewn on floors to ward off evil spirits.

King George VI was so impressed with this treatment for crushed fingers by the remedy he named his racehorse Hypericum. It won the English Classic race 'The 2000 Guineas' in 1947.

The mother tincture is prepared from the whole plant, which is a perennial herb with woody branches. The dotted leaves are opposite and the flowers deep yellow. The herb has a characteristic balsam odour and a bitter taste.

Keynotes

Nerve injuries especially fingers, toes and nails. Crushed fingers. Weakness of tendons and muscles. Lacerated painful wounds.

Therapeutic Duration

Fast – one day to one week (internally and externally).

Constitution

Practically no constitutional features (even Kent agrees!).

NOTE: Hypericum mother tincture blended in equal proportions with Calendula mother tincture is an excellent healant called *Hypercal*, when applied topically.

Modalities

> bending head backward > warm applications.
< cold < damp < closed rooms < exposure < touch < 3 to 4am < pressure.

Complementary Remedies

Ledum, Arnica.

Antidotes

Arsen alb., Chamomilla, Sulphur.

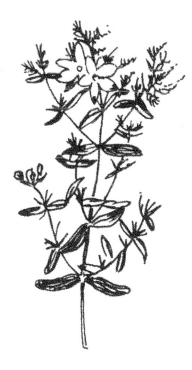

Hypericum perforatum

IGNATIA AMARA

Common names: St Ignatius' bean,
Strychnos ignatia
Abbreviation: Ignatia
Repertory abbreviation: Ign.

Source/Origin

Small tree with erect trunk and opposite branches. White flowers with the smell of jasmine (cf. Gelsemium). Pear-shaped fruit. Almond-shaped seeds are very hard and used to prepare the mother tincture. Bitter tasting. Indigenous to China and Philippines.

Proved by Hahnemann in 1805.

At the funeral of King George VI in 1952 in London, five Queens and three Kings were treated with Ignatia!

Keynotes

Hysteria. Grief, bereavement, pining. Mood swings. Sighing. Nervous headaches from worry. Twitching of facial muscles. Flatulence. Distended abdomen. Irritating cough.

Constitution

People with tendency to mood swings. Bright, precocious children and women who are very sensitive and nervous.

Gentle, sensitive, fine-fibred, highly educated, overwrought with nervous complaints (Kent).

They dislike meat and alcohol and tend to be jealous (cf. Lachesis).

Modalities

< stooping < morning < open air < after meals < coffee < smoking or tobacco smell < liquids < warmth < strong odours.
> while eating > change of position > sitting.
> pressure > summer.

Complementary Remedies

Natrum mur.

Antidotes

Pulsatilla (best antidote), Chamomilla, Cocculus.

IPECACUANHA

Caphaelis ipecacuanha

Common name: Ipecacuanha
Abbreviation: Ipecac.
Repertory abbreviation: Ip.

Source/Origin

The mother tincture is prepared from the whole, dried root of Ipecacuanha. A perennial plant with a partly buried stem up to 1m (3ft) long. Small white flowers. Dark brown root. Rhizome has peripheral vascular tissue. Contains the alkaloid *emetine*. Proved by Hahnemann (1805), *Allen's Encyclopedia*, Vol. V.

Keynotes

Acute conditions. Persistent nausea with vomiting. Leads all remedies for nausea (Nash). Cutting pains in stomach. Spasmodic conditions, e.g. asthma. Salivation. Violent, incessant cough with wheezing. Uterine haemorrhages. Menstrual problems. Diarrhoea. Whooping cough.

Constitution

Overweight children and adults. They may be irritable, anxious and very impatient but unsure for what. Inclined to sulk, complain about everything and hold everything in contempt (Kent).

Disdainful humour (Clarke).

Prone to colds, particularly in humid weather.

Modalities

< winter < lying down < emotional upset < periodically < moist, warm wind < food < motion < eating
> rest.

Complementary Remedies

Cuprum met.

Antidotes

Arsen alb., Cinchona, Tabacum, Arnica, Cinchona, Nux vomica.

IODUM

Common name: Iodine
Abbreviation: Iodum
Repertory abbreviation: Iod.

Source/Origin

The halogen element iodine, symbol I. Grey-black rhombic crystals. The remedy owes its importance primarily to the high iodine content of the hormone, *thyroxin*. Originally proved by Hahnemann, Allen's Encyclopedia, Vol. V.

Alternatively named Iodium.

Keynotes

Hypertrophy, enlarged glands (except mammary glands), especially lymphatic glands of abdomen and mesenteric glands. Restlessness, hunger (constant), thirst. Anxiety in mind and body. Feverish sweating. Emaciation. Grave's disease. (Overactive thyroid gland). Loss of memory. Lack of concentration. Weakness on exertion (ascending stairs).

Therapeutic Duration

About one month.

Constitution

Dark-haired thin people with dark skin, dark eyes and a staring look. Anxious when trying to keep still (Kent), but better for walking about.

Always hungry and wants to eat all the time and feels better for eating (Nash), yet gets thinner and thinner.

Glands are enlarged, nodular and hard (Tyler).

Depressed to the point of suicidal tendency, cannot contem-plate the future and wants to be alone. Young people who grow too rapidly.

Modalities

< cool room > eating > walking > open air < stooping < warm room < for silence < right side < night < ascending stairs.

Complementary Remedies

Kalium iodatum, Lycopodium, Badiaga.

Antidotes

Antim. tart., Apis mel., Arsen. alb., Aconite, Belladonna, China, Ferrum met., Graphites, Thuja, Sulphur.

KALIUM BICHROMICUM

Common names: Potassium dichromate, potassium bichromate
Abbreviation: Kali. bich.
Repertory abbreviation: Kali-bi

Source/Origin

Mineral with the formula $K_2Cr_2O_7$, potassium and chromium are both essential nutrients (see chapter 7). Orange, red transparent crystals or powder with a metallic taste. Corrosive, irritant poison.
'Stringy, spotty and yellow' (Tyler).

Keynotes

Special affinity for the mucous membranes especially in the respiratory tract. Thick discharges, especially from the nose. Arthritic disorders with moving symptoms. Asthma. Anaemia. Burning at root of nose with dryness and feeling of bone pressure (Tyler). Sinusitis. Thick, yellow, stringy, lumpy or ropy nasal discharges. Stomach disorders alternating with rheumatism or asthma.
NOTE: Periodicity – complaints may occur or be worse daily at a particular time.

Therapeutic Duration

Medium – one month.

Constitution

Fat, light-complexioned people who are inflexible and stick to a rigid routine. Tend to give long, elaborate answers to questions when a short answer would suffice. Will concentrate on his or her physical symptoms and ignore mental or emotional problems. Will become irritable and bad tempered with any material discomfort or denial.
A 'glucy' personality (Morrison).
Chilly people.

Modalities

< cold < morning < undressing < 1 to 2am (asthma)
> heat.

Complementary Remedies

Arsen alb., Hydrastis, Silica, other Kalium salts.

Antidotes

Arsen alb., Lachesis, Pulsatilla.

LACHESIS

Lachesis muta, Lachesis mutus

Common names: Bushmaster snake venom, Surucucu
Abbreviation: Lachesis
Repertory abbreviation: Lach.

Source/Origin

Important polycrest remedy.

The bushmaster snake inhabits hot areas in South America. Growing to more than 4m (12ft) long, its poison fangs are about 2.5cm (1in) long. Its skin is orange, reddish-brown, mottled with large black/brown spots. The venom is very poisonous and may be fatal. The remedy is prepared from the venom by stunning the snake and collecting on sugar by pressing the poison fang against the bag.
Proved by Constantine Hering in South America in 1828. (See Chapter 1).

Keynotes

Skin eruptions with coloration – bluish colour of surrounding skin and mottled appearance. Septic states. Menopausal problems (e.g. ovarian pain, left side). Delirium tremens with much trembling. Bursting, hammering (Kent) headaches. Vertigo, particularly on closing eyes. Intense photophobia – pain, itching, stinging and headache. Hoarseness (worse morning). Muscular spasms.

NOTE: Left-sided laterality, tending to the right side.

Therapeutic Duration

Medium – one month.

Constitution

Young, talkative person, furtive looking, with thin, unsmiling lips and glazed eyes. Quarrelsome and finding fault in everyone and everything. With lashing tongue, they do not realize the hurt they give. Cannot bear anything tight anywhere, such as about waist or around throat – always wants to tear at or loosen his or her collar. Prone to muscular spasms. Sheds tears of self-pity, not sympathy. Very jealous with suspicion (almost insane). Very sensitive to noise and prefers to be alone. May start suddenly from sleep. Best mental efforts are at night. Alternating moods with unbearable anxiety, particularly on waking, and gloom then fury. A poor sense of time.
For full constitution see Chapter 4.

Modalities

< after sleep < cold weather < motion < warm bath. < pressure < constriction (waist, throat) < touch
> discharges > warm applications > dark > swallowing solids > after eating.

Complementary Remedies

Crotalus, Acidum nit., Hepa., Sulph., Lycopodium.

Antidotes

Arsen alb., Mercurius sol., Natrum mur., Alumina, Belladonna, Cocculus, Coffea.

LEDUM PALUSTRE

Common names: Wild rosemary, marsh tea, marsh cistus
Abbreviation: Ledum
Repertory abbreviation: Led.

Source/Origin

Evergreen shrub growing up to 1m (3ft) in height with rust-coloured fir round branches. White or pale rose flowers with a bitter taste and strong aromatic odour. Indigenous to northern Europe, Asia and Canada. The whole plant is used to prepare the mother tincture. First proved by Hahnemann in 1805.

Keynotes

Punctured wounds by sharp, pointed instruments and wounds very sensitive to touch (Tyler).

Rheumatic diathesis, from feet upwards. Pain in knees. Skin eruptions. Antidote to insect stings (cf. Apis). All wounds are cold.

Therapeutic Duration

Medium – up to one month.

Constitution

Weak constitutionally. A very chilly, timid, anxious person. Lacking in animal vital heat and cold to the touch, particularly in the vicinity of wounds. The Ledum person seeks cold air (in spite of their coldness) and cold washing. Feet and hands, face and knees may be swollen, purple and sometimes mottled.

NOTE: Ledum is puffy, purple and cold (Lachesis is puffy, purple and hot).

Modalities

< lower limbs < evening and at night < heat of bed < cold < by covering.
> putting feet in cold water > application of iced water.

Complementary Remedies

Sepia.

Antidotes

Camphor, Coffea, Ipecacuanha, Rhus tox.

LYCOPODIUM CLAVATUM

Common name: Club moss
Abbreviation: Lycopodium
Repertory abbreviation: Lyc.

Source/Origin

Great polycrest remedy. Central to the entire *Materia Medica*. 'A knowledge of this remedy is essential to a proper understanding of the *Materia Medica*' (Clarke).

Perennial evergreen shrub with trailing, branching stem indigenous to Europe, Russia and North America. Pale yellow spores which are odourless and tasteless and form a fine mobile powder from which the mother tincture is prepared.

Proved by Hahnemann in 1828. 'This drug has real medicinal properties which can only be disclosed by trituration and succussion' (Hahnemann).

Keynotes

Action on the entire organism. Anxiety (before forthcoming events, cf. Argent nit.)). Asthma. Chronic fatigue syndrome. Painful skin eruptions – ulcers, abscesses. Constipation (long standing) with bloated, distended abdomen. Kidney stones (after Berberis). Irritable bowel syndrome (Morrison). Especially beneficial after Calc. carb. (Kent). Cramps in chest in stomach affections (Clarke).

Therapeutic Duration

Slow – six to eight weeks.

Constitution

Sickly looking, grey or balding person with yellowish-grey skin, thin and wrinkled, especially a frowning forehead but with heavy buttocks. Cheeks and nose may be red. Subject to nervous anticipation (cf. Argent nit. and Gelsemium), particularly when making a speech or giving a lecture or stage fright. Prefers to be alone but fears to be alone so likes a person in the next room. Fears crowds, darkness, death and people. Intellectual person but may make mistakes in writing and may select the wrong words in speaking. Lack of self-discipline.

Cowardice (Vithoulkas). Explosive temperament (like the spores from which it is derived). Not a constitution to stare one in the face, but after a few questions to the patient you will soon be hot on the trail (Tyler).

Modalities

< evening < right side < right to left < from above downwards < cold food and drink < 4 to 8pm < eating

> motion > after midnight > warm food > on becoming cold on being uncovered.

Complementary Remedies

Iodum, Lachesis, Pulsatilla, Ipecacuanha (bronchitis).

Antidotes

Aconite, Camphor, Causticum, Chamomilla, Graphites, Pulsatilla, Chelidonium. Coffea, Graphites, Nux vom.

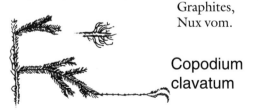

Copodium clavatum

MEDORRHINUM

Common name: Medorrhinum
Abbreviation: Medorrhinum
Repertory abbreviation: Med.

Source/Origin

Classic nosode prepared from the purulent discharge from an untreated case of gonorrhoea. Complex mixture of tissue and bacteria. Sexually transmitted disease involving the mucous membranes of the genito-urinary tract, rectum and cervix. A tubercular remedy with the beginnings of sycosis. Originally proved by Swan; *Materia Medica* of Nosodes, 1888.

Keynotes

Closely related to Thuja (sycotic miasm). Debility. Depression with anxiety. Discharges from genito-urinary tract. Irritation in genito-urinary tract (cf. Sycotic Co). Trembling – a state of collapse. Soft tissue tumours. Fluid retention. Pituitary dysfunction. Impotence.

Therapeutic Duration

Slow, deep seated.

Constitution

A weak, small, prematurely aged person with pallid, unhealthy skin and sluggish mind. Children are anaemic with large heads and sweaty faces, swollen glands and catarrh (cf. Baryta carb.). Warts, polyps and moles are common. The Medorrhinum person is always hurrying and worries. He or she is insecure, blushes easily, feels exhausted in the morning but is full of activity in the evening. Memory is poor. Sensitive and starts at the slightest sound. Chilly person. Craving for stimulants – alcohol, cigarettes, coffee, drugs.

Modalities

< thinking of complaints < touch < noise < draughts.
< cold weather < morning
> seaside > damp weather > lying on stomach > at night.

Complementary Remedies

Thuja, Natrum sulph., Argentum nit.

NATRUM MURIATICUM

Common name: Common salt, sodium chloride
Abbreviation: Nat. mur.
Repertory abbreviation: Nat-mur

Source/Origin

Produced by mining natural rock salt or the evaporation of sea water. Cubic, white crystals, granules or powder. Formula, NaCL. Proved by Hahnemann. *Hering's Guiding Symptoms*, Vol. VII.

Important polycrest remedy.

Keynotes

Weakness and exhaustion. Headache – blinding, school children. Colds – copious coryza, cough in mornings. Herpes of lips – corners and middle lower lip cracks. Hot and perspiring palms. Numbness and tingling in fingers. Coldness (whole body) with extreme chilliness. Nausea and stomach affections with capricious tastes and appetite. Oedema.

Therapeutic Duration

Slow – six to eight weeks.

Constitution

Yellowish skin with pale and earthy face. Tendency to pimples and dry, cracked lips. Sensitive teeth with tendency to mouth ulcers and bitter taste. Nurses grievances of family relations (cf. Sepia) and traumatic experiences and betrayal (Miss Havisham of Great Expectations – Coulter). Cannot bear sympathy of any kind and rejects physical closeness. Slow to learn to talk as a child. May be a 'tomboy'. Feeling dejected, isolated, lonely and desolate is common in depression. Bad tempered in the mornings and music saddens. Laughter his or her best antidote. Vulnerable, particularly to romantic love

Modalities

< sitting < bread < fat < wine < touch < morning < noise < warm room < music < lying down < 10am < seashore < mental exertion < sympathy < heat < talking < empty swallowing < toothache < coitus > lying on right side > open air > tight clothing > pressure (back).

Complementary Remedies

Arsen alb., Phosphorus, Nux vomica, Spig. nit. dulc.

NUX VOMICA

Common names: Poison nut (Strychnos nux vomica)
Abbreviation: Nux vom.
Repertory abbreviation: Nux-v

Source/Origin

Poison nut tree has a crooked, irregular trunk with smooth ash-coloured bark. Small, funnel-shaped green white flowers with disagreeable odour. Orange-yellow fruit, the size of an apple, containing five disc-shaped, bitter seeds.

Great polycrest remedy with many common symptoms of many common diseases. The poisonous seeds, which contain strychnine, are sometimes called 'Quakers' buttons', which is far removed from the Nux vomica-type lifestyle! They are used to prepare the mother tincture. Proved by Hahnemann, *Materia Medica* Pura, 3rd edn.

Keynotes

Spasmodic pain. Headache, *'the morning after'* hangover with (smoker's) cough.

Discharges from nostril or nostrils. Catarrhal headache. Coryza – sudden and violent. Gastric symptoms – biliousness, vomiting, colic. Haemorrhoids with blood in faeces. Diarrhoea/constipation. Frequent urination with burning and tearing pain. Flatulence. Alcoholism. Asthma.

Therapeutic Duration

Fast – up to one week.

Constitution

Thin, dark-haired, fast-moving, active, nervous individual. Particularly men, but also women in senior executive positions who are hypochondriacal. Never warm, particularly in bed. A driving 'goal-getter' placing production before people. Intelligent, ambitious, he (or she) seeks to achieve goals, impatient and get things done (cf. Arsen alb. who seeks perfection). Easily offended and competitive individual does not like to be contradicted. Bellicose, domineering and demanding, Nux vomica is a workaholic, staying long hours in the office. Suffers from mental strain and from his (or her) lifestyle – alcoholic stimulants, drinking copious quantities of coffee, rich business lunches, sex, smoking heavily and inadequate exercise. Catherine Coulter has suggested the character of Rhett Butler in *Gone with the Wind* as a typical Nux vomica type.

Modalities

< morning < mental exertion < after eating < stimulants (alcohol) < drugs < dry weather < cold < 3 to 4am (thinking of work next day). > after dozing > evening > wet weather > strong pressure.

Complementary Remedies

Sulphur, Kalium carb., Sepia.

Antidotes

Aconite, Belladonna, Camphor, Chamomilla, Coffea, Opium, Pulsatilla, Thuja, Euphorbium, Cocculus, Platina, Stramonium.

NOTE: Sepia follows well.

157

PETROLEUM

Common names: Petrol, gas, rock oil
Abbreviation: Petroleum
Repertory abbreviation: Petr.

Source/Origin

Crude oil, dark brown, green-black with characteristic odour. Density 0.77–0.87.

Proved originally with rectified oil by trituration by Hahnemann and subsequently reported by Constantine Hering, Guiding Symptoms, Vol. 8.

Important antipsoric remedy related to Graphites.

Keynotes

Skin – thick, green, crusty, itching, burning, raw with bleeding cracks (worse in winter). Irritable skin. Eczema. Herpes. Psoriasis. Diarrhoea. Vertigo on rising.

Catarrhal conditions of mucous membranes. Sea sickness. Car travel sickness.

Chilblains.

Therapeutic Duration

Slow – one to two months.

Constitution

Dark-skinned people with marked skin problems. Dry, cracked, leathery skin with unhealthy appearance. Cracked tips of fingers especially. Emotionally unstable and all conditions are worse in winter.

Modalities

< travelling (especially in cars, but also at sea) < winter < damp conditions < during and after thunderstorm.
< eating < open air < bathing.
> warmth > lying with head high > dry weather > dry weather > eating.

Complementary Remedies

Sepia.

Antidotes

Nux vomica, Cocculus.

PHOSPHORUS

Common name: Phosphorus
Abbreviation: Phosphorus
Repertory abbreviation: Phos.

Source/Origin

Colourless or pale yellow, translucent allotrope of the non-metallic element, phosphorus. Chemical symbol, P. Emits white fumes on exposure to air with garlic odour until totally vaporized. Ignites spontaneously when heated. Must be stored under water.

Proved by Hahnemann, Allen's *Encyclopedia Materia Medica*, Vol. 7 and The Chronic Diseases, 1st edn

Mother tincture prepared by melting phosphorus in hot alcohol.

Keynotes

Vertigo (particularly on rising quickly, turning the head or stooping). Migrainous headache. Deafness (own voice echoes). Nasal catarrh (with red, shiny nose). Hard, dry cough. Dry, scaly skin eruptions, e.g. dandruff. Psoriasis. Stiffness in limbs (< morning). Corpulence. Smoking habit.

NOTE: Feeling of intense heat up back.

Therapeutic Duration

Slow – up to six weeks.

Constitution

Tall, slender, narrow-chested persons with thin, transparent, waxy looking skin, fair or red-haired, fine hair and delicate eyelashes. Emaciated appearance.

Intelligent people with artistic flair and thin, tapered hands. Anaemic with pink or white complexion. Over-sensitive to environment, such as light, sound, smells and touch. Difficulties with other people in their neighbourhood. Liable to be aggressive even to the point of (but not actual) violence, followed quickly by remorse. Flushes easily when embarrassed or excited. Fast-growing young people who tend to stoop. Faddish about foods and must eat often or gets a sinking, empty feeling in abdomen. Ethereal personality with spasmodic brilliance.

Modalities

< touch < physical or mental exertion < warm food.
< warm drinks < getting wet < noise < ascending stairs.
> in dark > lying on right side > cold food and drinks.
> sleep > open air > during thunderstorm.

Complementary Remedies

Arsen alb., Cepa, Lycopodium, Silicea, Sanguinaria, Carbo veg.

Antidotes

Nux vomica, Causticum, Terebinthum, Kalium permanganum.

PSORINUM

Common name: Scabies vesicle
Abbreviation: Psorinum
Repertory abbreviation: Psor.

Source/Origin

Import nosode of the psoric miasm. Hahnemann's first nosode of diseased material, published in Stapf's Archives, 1833. Prepared from the sero-purulent matter of the scabies vesicle.

Useful in chronic cases when the remedy selected according to the Simillimum fails to cure.

Keynotes

Lack of vital reaction. Strong affinity for the skin. Skin eruptions, raw, bleeding fissures, eruptions around fingernails. Boils, pimples, oozing sores. Raw, itching, weeping eczema. Intolerable itching. Asthma (< lying down with arms apart). Offensive discharges.

NOTES: 200C potency and higher is preferred. Psorinum features strongly in the '*Never been well since…*' syndrome.

Therapeutic Duration

Slow – thirty to forty days (may take up to nine days before therapeutic action manifests itself).

Constitution

Scrofulous person with long nose, pale, delicate complexion, coarse, dirty, tawny coloured skin, sweating profusely with body odour. Hair is dry, lustreless, tangles easily and sticks together (Hering). Can be very depressed with suicidal tendencies. They believe they will never recover from any illness. Pessimistic in the extreme. Offensive discharges with oozing scabs and intolerable itching. Sweaty feet with fetid odour and eruptions around fingernails. Very sensitive to cold, wanting warm clothing even in summer and the head kept warm. Lack of vital heat. Often hungry with desire to eat in the night – raiding the refrigerator. 'Canine hunger' (Kent) for junk food. Still look dirty and smelly even after washing. If Sulphur represents the great unwashed, Psorinum represents the great unwashable (Roberts).

NOTE: In modern society with better hygiene the features described above are generally less severe.

Modalities

< coffee < changes of weather < hot sunshine < cold < cold draft < before thunderstorm < winter.
> heat > warm clothing > when eating.

Complementary Remedies

Sulphur, Bacillinum.

Antidotes

Coffea.

PULSATILLA NIGRICANS

Common names: Wind flower, meadow anemone
Abbreviation: Pulsatilla
Repertory abbreviation: Puls.

Source/Origin

Fascinating, pre-eminently female, polycrest remedy. Recently affinity for homosexual males demonstrated.

A perennial plant with a thin, simple, rounded, erect stem. Dark violet to light blue bell-shaped, pendulous flowers, growing in clumps in open fields and meadows, all over Europe, Russia and Asia.

Proved by Hahnemann in 1805 (*Encyclopedia Materia Medica*, Vol. 8). The mother tincture is prepared from the whole fresh plant. Called the '*wind flower*' as its thin stem readily bends with the wind.

Keynotes

Headaches, migraines (particularly at end of periods). Vertigo. Sore throat with dryness (yet no thirst). Hay fever. Wandering pains. Difficult menstruation – easily suppressed, short, irregular and changeable flow. Dysmenorrhea at puberty. Measles. Asthma. Greenish, thick nasal discharges. Conjunctivitis. Itching and lachrymation. Catarrh. Rheumatism. Cramping abdominal and womb pains. Pre-menstrual headaches and tender breasts. Hahnemann said, '*Even the smallest medicine chest should contain Pulsatilla*'.

Therapeutic Duration

Slow – up to four weeks.

Constitution

Mainly females, probably a teenager, with fair or blonde hair and blue eyes. A shy, gentle, good-natured disposition, yielding to the slightest pressure and afraid of the dark (fears ghosts). Romantic, emotional, crying readily with tendency to inward grief (Tyler). A changeable, moody person yielding to pressure from others. Person liable to depression. Chilly yet seeks open, cool air. Hates stuffy rooms. Sleeps with one pillow and hands over head or one over head and the other under the pillow and bedroom window open. Special affinity for slow, phleg-matic temper-aments (Tyler). Pulsatilla women are very responsive to sympathy (opposite of Natrum mur.) – need support and reassurance. Dislikes butter and fatty foods. '*Will hide behind her mother's skirts when a stranger appears then slowly emerges with a smile*' (Hahnemann).

Modalities

< during periods < heat < rich, fat food, butter, pork < late afternoon < left side < allowing feet to hang down < sitting (vertigo and backache) < sun < warmth.

> open air > motion > cold applications > cold food and drinks > tight bandaging > sitting upright > rubbing hard > lying on painful side.

Complementary Remedies

Acid sulph., Lycopodium, Allium cepa, Silicea, Kali. sulph., Stannum met., Kali. mur.

Antidotes

Asafoetida, Coffea, Chamomilla, Ignatia, Nux vomica, Stannum met., Calc. phos.

RHUS TOXICODENDRON

Common names: Poison ivy, poison oak
Abbreviation: Rhus tox.
Repertory abbreviation: Rhus

Source/Origin

A major polycrest remedy, poison ivy is a deciduous shrub with reddish branching stems growing up to 1m (3ft) in height. Large green leaves are pointed. Small greenish-white flowers. Extremely poisonous with numbness and tingling when touching the leaves. So poisonous a licence is required to grow it. Sometimes called 'the *Rusty Gate*'.

Keynotes

Rheumatic pain, joints, tendons, etc. Affections of mucous membranes. Strains. Septic conditions. Inflammations becoming pustular. Sciatic, pain.
NOTE: The lowest permissible potency prescribed is 3X.

Therapeutic Duration

Fast – one to seven days.

Constitution

Weak constitutionally. The Rhus tox. type of person is listless, depressed and extremely restless, wanting constantly to 'limber up' and change position. Subject to rheumatic pains with stiffness. Always feeling worse at night with nervous apprehension and wants to get up and walk about.

Modalities

< during sleep < cold wet weather < after rain at night < during rest < lying on back < lying on right side.
> warm > dry weather > motion (but worse on initial motion)
> walking > change of position > rubbing > warm applications > stretching out limbs.

Complementary Remedies

Bryonia, Calc. carb., Calc. fluor., Phytolacca.

Antidotes

Anarcardium, Aconite, Ammon. Carb., Belladonna, Bryonia, Camphor, Coffea, Clematis, Croton tig., Graphites, Grindelia, Lachesis, Ranun. bulb., Sulphur, Sepia.

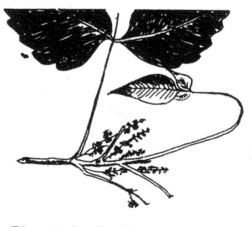

Rhus toxicodendron

RUTA GRAVEOLENS

Common names: Rue, Herb of Grace, Rue Bitterwort
Abbreviation: Ruta grav.
Repertory abbreviation: Ruta

Source/Origin

Perennial herb from Southern Europe with grey-green leaves and bright yellow flowers with four petals set wide apart, growing in dry, shady places and disliking cold and wet conditions (see Modalities). It has a strong scent and a bitter taste ('Rue – sour' 'Herb of Grace', Richard III, Shakespeare). Strewn on floors in ancient times as a prophylactic against pestilence or plague.

The mother tincture is prepared from the whole fresh plant just before the flowers develop. Proved by Hahnemann, *Materia Medica Pura*, Vol. IV.

Keynotes

Bruised, injured bones (cf. Arnica). Sprains, strained sore tendons. Painful joints, muscular pain. Eyestrain from reading or fine work (followed by headache). Anal prolapse, piles after frequent, unsuccessful urging. Sciatica.

Compares with Rhus toxicodendron in many features.

Therapeutic Duration

Medium – up to one month.

Constitution

Tired-looking person with watery, red eyes and no other particular facial features. Restless, not wanting to sit for any length of time (Gibson). Tendency to flop back when rising from a chair. Unsteady gait with stiffness of limbs. Anxious feelings, peevishness and tendency to contradict and pick quarrels. May weep out of annoyance over recent actions, but not in repentance.

Modalities

< cold < wet < rest < lying down < walking outdoors < fixed look at objects < touch < stooping < raw food < during periods.
> warmth > moving indoors > pressure > lying on back.

Complementary Remedies

Calc. phos., Silicea.

Antidotes

Camphor.

SEPIA OFFICINALIS

Common name: Ink or juice of cuttlefish, squid
Abbreviation: Sepia
Repertory abbreviation: Sep.

Source/Origin

The cuttlefish is a mollusc without an external shell, 30–60cm (1–2ft) long of soft, gelatinous body. The mouth is surrounded by ten arms furnished with suckers. The ink is an excreting liquid contained in a bag or sac within the abdomen. It is a blackish, brown pigment and is discharged into the water when the cuttlefish is threatened or about to attack its prey. The inky juice from which the mother tincture is prepared by trituration has been used by artists as a brown pigment for centuries. Proved by Hahnemann, 1828.

Keynotes

Uterine dysfunctions. Flatulence with headache. Pain from below upwards. Sensation of a ball in the rectum. Cystitis. Prolapsed uterus, vagina or rectum.

Therapeutic Duration

Slow – one to two months.

Constitution

Especially in women, the Sepia type has a yellowish complexion with blonde or red hair and a saddle-like yellow, brownish band across nose and cheeks. They walk with a stoop and sit with crossed legs fearing a prolapsed uterus or vagina. They are indifferent to loved ones and family. They are depressed and irritable, easily offended and hate to be alone. They always feel cold even in a warm room, and are indolent and mean.

Modalities

< morning and evening < damp < left side < sweating < cold air < before thunderstorm < moving arms.
> exercise > pressure > warmth in bed > cold bathing.
> after sleep.

Complementary Remedies

Nux vomica, Natrum mur. and other Natrum salts, Sabadilla.

Antidotes

Aconite, Antim crud., Antim tart., Sulphur, Rhus tox.

SILICEA

Common names: Silica, flint, sandstone, silicon dioxide, silicic anhydride
Abbreviation: Silica
Repertory abbreviation: Sil.

Source/Origin

White amorphous (no crystalline form) powder which is tasteless and odourless. Silicon dioxide, formula SiO_2. Mother tincture prepared in solid form by trituration as the oxide is insoluble in alcohol/water solutions. May be converted to liquid potencies at 8X and above.

Keynotes

Prolonged sick headache with nausea and perhaps vomiting. Styes. Dyslexia. Hardened glands, especially around neck. Cold, clammy sweat on forehead, yet lower part of body is dry and cold. Warty growths. Moist eruptions. Suppurative conditions (cf. Hepar sulph.). Constipation during periods. Sleeplessness with nightwalking. Ill effects of vaccination (cf. Thuja). As if *'hair on tongue'* (sensation).

Therapeutic Duration

Slow – two to three months.

Constitution

Faint-hearted, yielding persons who are nervous and excitable. Lack grit (Tyler). Weak, embarrassed easily. Chilly person lacking stamina. He or she dreads failure, particularly with a mental task to perform, but performs well. Irritable, irascible when aroused but when alone individual is mild, gentle and tearful – complementing Pulsatilla (Kent). Depressed and despondent, dreading undertaking anything.

Modalities

< draughts < alcohol < winter < cold, damp weather < after bath < mental exertion (headache).
> wrapping up > summer.

Complementary Remedies

Calc. carb., Pulsatilla, Thuja, Sanicula.

Antidotes

Camphor, Hepar sulph., Acid fluor.

STAPHYSAGRIA

Common names: Stavesacre, Delphinium Staphysagria
Abbreviation: Staphysagria
Repertory abbreviation: Staph.

Source/Origin

Annual herb with large root and light blue flowers. The fruit hangs in three oblong capsules holding about twelve seeds in two rows. The powdered seed is used to prepare the mother tincture of the remedy. Introduced by Hahnemann in 1819.

Keynotes

Eczema. Bladder irritation (cf. Cantharis). Lacerated tissues. Sensation of dripping urine along genito-urinary tract. Frequent urge to urinate. Pain with stiffness in calf muscles. Prostate affections. Toothache. Flatulent colic.

Therapeutic Duration

Medium – up to one month.

Constitution

Over-sexed, very sensitive people with sunken eyes, liable to violent, passionate outbursts. Very sensitive to verbal insults, showing much anger. Often heavy smokers. Marked irritability.

Modalities

< anger < indignation < grief < sexual excess touch < dehydration < tobacco < sitting < coitus (men).
> warmth > after breakfast > rest at night.

Complementary Remedies

Causticum, Colocynthis.

Antidotes

Ambra gris, Camphor.

SULPHUR

Common name: Sulphur
Abbreviation: Sulphur
Repertory abbreviation: Sulph.

Source/Origin

Known as 'the *Common Denominator*'. A major antipsoric polycrest that sits astride the entire homoeopathic *Materia Medica*. A mainstay remedy. More proving symptoms than any other remedy. Known as a remedy for two thousand years.

Fine yellow powder of the element sulphur (sulfur – USA). Chemical symbol, S. Sulphur burns with a blue flame and melts to a dark red liquid at 115°C (239°F), with offensive characteristic odour.

Introduced by Hahnemann, *Allen's Encyclopedia*, Vol. 9 and *The Chronic Diseases*, Vol. 2.

Keynotes

Skin affections with burning heat and smarting. Skin eruptions with itching and redness (acne, eczema)(may alternate with asthma). Constipation. Dizziness, particularly on standing. Halitosis. Conditions which suggest no obvious indications for a partic-ular remedy. It is often said that if you repertorize long enough you will usually end up with Sulphur! Sulphur frequently raises therapeutic power when other remedies fail to act.

Therapeutic Duration

Slow – six to eight weeks.

Constitution

Warm-blooded people with coarse hair, yellowish skin, red ears, flush easily with red, sweaty palms. Body orifices, lips, etc. may be bright red and there may be body odour. Prone to skin problems and very thirsty (guzzles!, cf. Arsenalb.). Untidily dressed, unkempt, unwashed with dirty finger nails. Sulphur types are intellectual with a poor memory (especially names) and a need for personal recognition ('*I cured that patient*', not '**Arnica** *cured that patient*'). They are chauvinistic, indifferent to the welfare of others. Argumentative, provocative, impatient but act as a catalyst in a group activity. Heated emotional outbursts and liable to depression. A nature of extremes, for example, selfish but occasional generosity or active then lazy. Sulphur types like short naps. '*We are all at one time or another in life Sulphur types*'. (Coulter).

Modalities

< winter < at rest < washing < looking down < before storms < 11am < warmth in bed < morning < cold < open air < from stooping < periodically < for alcohol < wet, damp < severe cold.
> drawing up limbs > warm weather > lying on right side > dry.

Complementary Remedies

Aconite, Arsen alb., Aloe, Badiaga, Nux vomica (at night), Psorinum, Sulphur (morning).

Antidotes

Aconite, Camphor, Arsen alb., Cinchona, Conium mac., Causticum, Nux vomica, Pulsatilla, Rhus tox, Sepia, Silicea, Chamomilla, Merc sol., Iodum, Acidum nit, Thuja.

SYMPHYTUM OFFICINALE

Common names: Comfrey, Knitbone, Bone set.
Abbreviation: Symphytum
Repertory abbreviation: Symph.

Source/Origin

Perennial herb with thick roots in tubers. White-yellow or purple flowers. Indigenous to UK and US. The mother tincture is prepared from the dried powdered root. Introduced into homoeopathy by Crosemo in 1887. Named 'knitbone' by the Ancients who recognized the power of the root in the treatment of non-union of bone fractures.

Keynotes

Bone fractures. Speeds up union of bone tissues. Pricking pains. Joint injuries. Skin healant. Eye pain following blow by blunt instrument. Duodenal ulcers (cf. Proteus and Dys co.). Backache from sexual excess. Sore breasts. Eye injuries. Sprains.

Constitution

Weak constitutionally. Feels as if ears stopped up.

Modalities

< pressure > rest.

Complementary Remedies

Calc phos.

Antidotes

None listed.

NOTE: Arnica follows well.

TARAXACUM

Taraxacum officinalis

Common names: Leontodum taraxacum, dandelion, puff ball
Abbreviation: Taraxacum
Repertory abbreviation: Tarax.

Source/Origin

Deciduous, perennial herb with long, cylindrical, tapering root. The shiny green leaves (sometimes eaten in salads) have sharp, unequally toothed lobes pointing down-wards. The bright golden-yellow flowers open to sunny weather in April to September. The whole plant contains a milky juice. Found in the northern hemisphere.

The root, lifted in the autumn, is used for the mother tincture.

Keynotes

Diuretic. Bitter taste in mouth with salivation. Profuse night sweats. Mapped tongue (leaves red sore patches when scraped) with white coating or brown coating in morning. Gallstones. Bilious attacks. Cold fingertips and hands and nose cold at 8pm.

Therapeutic Duration

Medium – two to three weeks.

Constitution

Weak constitutionally. The Taraxacum type is loquacious (cf. Lachesis) and inclined to laugh but lacks resolution and avoids work. Liable to have cold hands and fingertips. Giddiness with vertigo may be frequent and gastric and bilious attacks with flatulence. There may be aversion to light. Several sensations: as if larynx were compressed, as if bubbles forming and bursting in abdomen.

Modalities

< at night < rest < lying down < sitting
> by touch > open air > by drinking > moving.

Complementary Remedies

None listed.

Antidotes

Camphor.

TARANTULA HISPANICA

Common names: Lycosa tarantula, Wolf spider, Spanish spider
Abbreviation: Tarantula
Repertory abbreviation: Tarant.

Source/Origin

The mother tincture is prepared from the live Spanish spider found in Spain and Italy. A vicious-looking spider whose venom affects the motor and sensory functions of the nervous system, resulting in a bizarre manic behaviour of the person bitten with excitability, excessive sensitivity and seizures of exhibitionism, nymphomania and dancing mania. The latter gave rise to the Spanish dance called the '*Tarentella*'.

Keynotes

Psychological disturbance with perpetual motion. Hysteria. Violence. Destructiveness. Extreme restlessness. Vertigo. Headaches with photophobia (right pupil may be enlarged). Chronic coryza with frequent sneezing and spasmodic cough. Constriction when swallowing (cf. Lachesis). Cystitis.

Therapeutic Duration

Fast.

Constitution

Pale-faced person with earthy look and wide, staring eyes suggesting terror. Throbbing carotids in neck. Constantly moving – jerking, twitching, dancing. Hands and fingers are never still. Can be very destructive. Constantly picks at fingers and screws up bits of paper before throwing them away. Constantly changing symptoms from excessive fits of laughter and singing, followed by deep depression. Cunning yet timid with a sly, furtive destructiveness. Flies into a rage when contradicted. Very sensitive to music – excited by musical rhythms.

Modalities

< strong emotion < music < cold < damp < walking < noise < light < wetting hands in cold water < rest < after sleep < night < after sexual intercourse.
> music > dry, sunny weather > open air > after nosebleed > warm room > pressure > friction.

Complementary Remedies

Agaricus, Arsen alb., Cuprum met., Mag. phos.

Antidotes

Lachesis.

THUJA OCCIDENTALIS

Common name: Arbor vitae, Tree of Life, white cedar
Abbreviation: Thuja
Repertory abbreviation: Thuj.

Source/Origin

Evergreen conifer growing to a small tree. The tree is tapered and the wood is fragrant like aromatic honey. Distinctive cones. The mother tincture is prepared from the fresh twigs.

A polycrest remedy characterized by its affinity for epithelial tissue.

Proved by Hahnemann, *Materia Medica Pura*, Vol. 5.

Keynotes

Skin eruptions. Warts on hands, fingers, face and ano-genital region. Ill-effects of vaccination. Flatulence with distended abdomen. Emaciation. Conjunctivitis with eyelids stuck together in morning. Precursors of chronic conditions with Thuja are suppressed gonorrhoea (sycotic), suppressed warts (psoric) and vaccination.

Therapeutic Duration

Slow – up to two months.

Constitution

Dark haired, probably male person with low self-esteem and feeling of worthlessness (Gray). Thick-set person with short neck, with reddish face and skin of honey-like aromatic odour, oily perspiration and possible warts on hands, fingers, face or eyelids. May have brown spots on face and arms and brittle nails (cf. Graphites). Very chilly with icy hands and cold knees and feet in bed. The Thuja patient is often called (like the remedy) 'the *Masquerader*' on account of their elusive, contradictory nature, never quite what they seem to be.

Modalities

< night < from heat of bed < 3am < 3pm < cold, damp air < after breakfast < after vaccination.
> left side > drawing up limb.

Complementary Remedies

Sabina, Arsen alb., Natrum sulph., Silicea.

Antidotes

Merc sol., Camphor, Sabina, Pulsatilla, Cocculus, Sulphur, Staphysagria, Chamomilla.

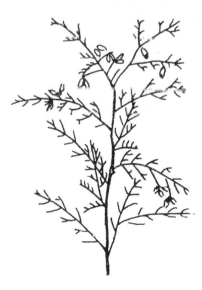

Thuja occidentalis

TUBERCULINUM

Common names: Tuberculinum, bacillinum (Dr Burnett), tuberculinum borinum
Abbreviation: Tuberculinum
Repertory abbreviation: Tub.

Source/Origin

Nosode of tubercular miasm. Tubercular glands of slaughtered cattle (Kent). Cultured bacilli from human tubercular tissue. The 30th centesimal potency is usually prescribed (not lower potencies).

Keynotes

Incipient pulmonary tuberculosis. Headache with periodicity. Constipation. Epilepsy. Neurasthenia. Trembling. Arthritis. Tonsilitis.

NOTE:
1. Needs frequent repetition in children's conditions, otherwise infrequent (Tyler).
2. Great value when symptoms are changing constantly, when well-selected remedies fail to improve symptoms and when colds result from slightest exposure.

3. Syphilinum follows Tuberculinum well.

Constitution

Pale-complexioned, blonde, blue eyed with bluish pallor. Narrow-chested people who recuperate slowly from any condition. They are always tired and avoid work (mental or physical) and like to travel. They are very sensitive and susceptible to changes in the weather and take cold on the least exposure. Mentally deficient children or children with temper tantrums. They may be depressed, anxious and irritable, inclined to sulk and have a fear of dogs.

Modalities

< music < before a storm < damp < draught < early morning < after sleep < initial motion then better on continuing (cf. Rhus tox.).
> open air > cold milk > sweets (candies).

Complementary Remedies

Psorinum, Hydrastis, Sulphur, Belladonna, Calc. carb.

VERATRUM ALBUM

Common name: White hellebore
Abbreviation: Veratrum alb.
Repertory abbreviation: Verat.

Source/Origin

Member of the lilac family of plants. Perennial herb with an erect rhizome, sometimes divided into branches, indigenous to the entire European continent. White-yellow flowers. The rhizome is used to prepare the mother tincture. Known to the ancient Greeks for its healing power, Veratrum album was the subject of Hahnemann's dissertation, presented in Latin, Greek and German in the Grand Hall of the University of Leipzig in 1812, given in order to gain a professorial post.

Keynotes

Collapse (cf. Carbo veg.). Cramp in calves (cf. Cuprum). Voracious appetite followed by vomitting. Bulimia. Constipation with large stools, particularly babies, when cold. May be followed by diarrhoea. Post-operative shock. Dryness and burning. Icy coldness. Copious discharges.

Therapeutic Duration

Medium – up to one month.

Constitution

A quarrelsome person who is pessimistic about the future and always cold. Cold, bluish skin (cf. Carbo veg.) with pinched features and cold perspiration on the forehead with most ailments.

Modalities

< cold < night < wet weather < least motion < touch.
> walking > warmth > pressure.

Complementary Remedies

Arnica.

Antidotes

Aconite, Arsen alb., Camphor, Cinchona, Coffea.

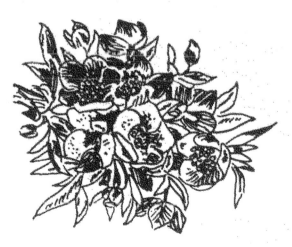

Veratrum album

ZINCUM METALLICUM

Common name: Zinc metal
Abbreviation: Zincum
Repertory abbreviation: Zinc

Source/Origin

Bluish white, lustrous metal. Symbol, Zn. Prepared by trituration of the powdered metal with lactose (USP or BP) to 7X and thence by liquid potentization to 8X and higher. Essential micro-nutrient. Alloyed with copper for brass. Somewhat neglected but now being used more widely. Proved by Hahnemann, Allen's Encyclopedia, Vol. X.

Keynotes

Anaemia. Mental and physical exhaustion. Lethargy. Depression. Restlessness (particularly feet). Spinal pain (dorsal and lumbar). Varicose veins (legs). Constipation. Poor memory. Alcoholism.

Therapeutic Duration

Medium – one month.

Constitution

Pale-faced, anaemic people who are nervous, lazy and lethargic. Hypochondriacal. Irascible and impatient. They are very sensitive to noise and uncommunicative. Mental and physical exhaustion. Strong dislike of wine and east fast. Children tend to repeat everything said to them.

Modalities

< touch < during period < 5 to 7pm < after dinner < wine < mental emotion < sitting (spine).
> when eating > discharges.

Complementary Remedies

Calc. phos.

Antidotes

Camphor, Hepar sulph., Ignatia.

CHAPTER 9
Applied Homoeopathy

*Polypharmacy. Bowel nosodes. Biotherapies –
organotherapy, lithotherapy, gemmotherapy.
Allergens. Homoeopathic drainage therapy.*

INTRODUCTION

Combination remedies are anathema to
classical homoeopaths. Allergens as
homoeopathic prophylactics are considered
by some homoeopaths to be inappropriate.
The biotherapies are based on clinical data
and not on Hahnemann's provings. The
Bach flower remedies are considered by many
homoeopaths not to be homoeopathic. As a
result, none of these remedies are included in
the homoeopathic *Materia Medicas* or the
Repertories, although some merit mention in
the appendices of the homoeopathic
Pharmacopoeias.

These views are widespread among
homoeopaths and are so contentious that
these so-called 'modern' aspects of
homoeopathy are often ignored in the
literature. However, homoeopathy must not
become monolithic and new approaches or
ideas must at least be aired freely and given
proper consideration. Every scientific and
technological discipline recognizes *'pure'*
and *'applied'* facets, for example pure and
applied mathematics. For this reason I have
called these aspects **applied** homoeopathy.

In the interests of the teaching of
homoeopaths across a whole, broad
spectrum, I believe this applied homoeopathy is worthy of discussion and it is for
fully informed, discerning students to form
their own opinions.

POLYPHARMACY

Polypharmacy is defined as the preparation
and prescription of combinations or
mixtures of two or more homoeopathic
remedies. Hahnemann, of course, taught the
classical prescription of the single remedy
only, chosen according to the Similimum.
He did not rule against the use of more than
one remedy, but *not at the same time.*

The basic concept of the combination
remedy is that the product represents the
sum of the proving symptoms of the
constituent remedies. Proponents of
combination remedies claim that they address
the need to cover the totality of symptoms.

The assumption, therefore, is that they act
synergistically, although regrettably some
commercial combinations include remedies
that antidote one another, for example, a
combination of Arsenicum album and Nux
vomica, although sharing a wide range of
similar symptoms is not viable since these
remedies mutually antidote one another.

The number of remedies in combinations produced by the manufacturers ranges from seven to thirty. It is thought that more extensive mixtures become counter-productive.

Clearly a **combination remedy is not appropriate for the treatment of a chronic disease**. If combinations are effective, it is in the sphere of acute diseases where pathological symptoms predominate. It follows, therefore, that they should be prescribed only for superficial, acute symptoms in low potencies, commonly 3X, 6X or 12X or 6C and, sometimes, even including mother tinctures. A variation called a Homaccord includes a range of potencies of each constituent remedy in the combination. It is believed that thereby they provide therapeutic action in a continuous flow – the next higher potency becoming available as the lower potency is exhausted.

Homoeopathic combination remedies are stocked in many pharmacies and health stores. Sold over the counter, the label carries an indication, for example 'For the Relief of Rheumatic Pain' or 'Indigestion Tablets'. Whether we accept combination remedies or not, they are quite popular with the general public and when purchased over the counter they can serve as an introduction to homoeopathy for minor ailments and often lead the user to seek homoeopathic treatment by a trained practitioner for more serious conditions.

BOWEL NOSODES

Although bowel nosodes are based on clinical evidence only, such was the reputation, experience and integrity of Dr Edward Bach and Dr John Paterson and his wife Elizabeth, and the fact that their painstaking research extended to no less than twelve thousand cases, they are now generally accepted in mainstream homoeopathy.

Bowel nosodes are homoeopathic medicines derived from potentized cultures of human stools containing intestinal bacteria and bacteria on the walls of the intestinal tract.

Dr Paterson explained their action in his paper published in the *British Homoeopathic Journal* in 1936 entitled 'The Potentized Drug and its Action on the Bowel Flora'.

B. coli and coliform organisms found in the intestinal tracts of all warm-blooded animals are non-pathogenic and harmless in the healthy bowel. Their role is to break up complex organic substances formed in the digestive processes into more simple substances to prepare them for normal excretion from the body.

The bowel microflora in the adult are highly variable and homoeopathic prescriptions can only be reliably based on Paterson's symptomatology. They serve many important functions, as defined by Williams (1996):

1. Providing a continuous low level response from the immune system and in the turnover and differentiation of intestinal epithelial tissue.
2. Providing a barrier to infection by enteric pathogens, by acid production, spatial exclusion, substrate competitition, bacteriocin production and deconjugation of bile acids.
3. Providing a source of nutrients, such as B vitamins, fatty acids and amino acids.
4. Providing enzyme augmentation.
5. Detoxification of many substances including some modern drugs.

When the body becomes diseased Bach and Paterson observed that the B. coli modify

Lithotherapy

Dr Bergeret and Dr Tetau have been primarily responsible for this new branch of homoeopathy in research programmes carried out in France in the 1970s and 1980s.

Lithotherapy may be defined as the use of homoeopathic remedies prepared from selected naturally occurring mineral rocks. It aims to re-establish the required levels of essential mineral and trace element nutrients in the body by the chemical process of dechelation.

The importance of the metals calcium, copper, cobalt, lithium, manganese, chromium, molybdenum, vanadium and the metalloid selenium, as essential nutrients and their activity on certain enzymes in the body, is now well documented (see Chapter 7, *The Twelve New Cell Salts*). However, patients with any diseases related to a deficiency of these minerals nevertheless showed the body content to be quite normal in analysis of their blood serum. For example, calcium and phosphorus levels in cases of osteoporosis were found to be normal, when the symptoms of this disease are known to rise from a deficiency. Assuming a proper dietary intake of these minerals, then, it may be assumed that there is a blockage or entrapment whereby, although the minerals are present in sufficient quantities, they are not available for utilization in the body's metabolism. Lithotherapy aims to restore the availability of these essential minerals by normalizing metabolic pathways disturbed by blockage at enzyme level. Enzyme deficiencies are of two types, the first being due to their absence in the body due to hereditary deficiencies and the second through inactivation of the necessary enzyme by the absence of essential metallic ions.

Increasing the amount of alimentary intake of these metals and metalloids simply causes the body to react by rejecting the excess quantities. Increased pollution of the environment with the inhalation of sulphur products and traces of pesticides, as well as chelating agents in antibiotics, analgesics and diuretics, results in an excessive intake.

Chemically the blocking of metal ions is the result of the process of chelation. In this process a free metal ion (positively charged) receives two pairs of electrons (negatively charged) donated by two nitrogen atoms in a protein-type molecule. The donor molecule 'grips' the metal ion rather like the claws of a crab and prevents it carrying out its essential role in the body's metabolism (*chele* is the Greek word for a crab's claw).

It is believed that the dechelating action of lithotherapy arises from an analogy between the crystalline structures of the chelated compound and the natural mineral rocks from which the remedies are prepared. For example, the natural rock Feldspar with a quadratic (four-sided) crystalline structure, rather than the triclinic (six-sided) crystalline structure, is effective in the treatment of osteoporosis.

Some lithotherapeutic remedies with th clinical indications are:

Apatite (Calcium, fluorine phosphorus) = Rheumatism
Barytine (Barium) = Dry and weeping eczema
Haematite (Iron) = Anaemia
Lepidolite (Lithium) = Depression
Rhodonite (Manganese, silicon) = Insomnia

DOSAGE: Lithotherapy is normally prescribed in an 8X potency only. This potency was selected as it is the lowest potency that can exist in liquid form for the very insoluble mineral rocks employed. The recommended dosage is ten drops on the tongue once daily. A course of treatment may extend from two to three months.

NOTE: There is a positive aspect of chelation in that it may be employed to counter toxic metal poisoning. For example, EDTA (ethylene diamine tetramine) is used for the treatment of cadmium or chromium poisoning.

Gemmotherapy

Gemmotherapeutic remedies are unique in that they represent the only example of a solvent other than alcohol and water being used in their potentization, namely glycerin. A typical mixture may be 20 per cent alcohol (v/v), 40 per cent water (v/v) and 40 per cent glycerine (v/v).

The sources of the remedies are the fresh buds, young shoots, rootlets or any embryonic tissue in the growth phase of plants, shrubs or trees. These sources are rich in chemical growth substances, such as vitamins, minerals and trace elements, auxins, anthocyanins, and flavenenoids, which it is believed provide a natural basis for highly active remedies. Flavenoids have a particular function in countering the formation of the free radicals believed to cause cell damage.

Flavenoids have recently been associated with a lower risk of heart attack. Dr Quinlan at the Royal Society of Medicine has claimed that flavenoids are important in neutralizing free radicals – which build up as toxins that attack the body cells eventually leading to heart disease, cancer and strokes. The toxins are caused by pollution, smoking and even sunlight. 'Each cell in the body takes 10,000 hits per day, a huge amount of damage occurs within the body and one of our best defences against these components are antioxidants like flavenoids which neutralize toxins.'

Clinical research carried out in France since 1965 has demonstrated that gemmotherapeutic remedies, like the sarcodes, have an affinity for specific organs or tissues in the body and specific indications for their use is possible. For example, *Ribes nigrum* (buds of blackcurrant) has a marked analgesic effect in all rheumatic conditions and *Sequoia gigantea* (buds of the California Sequoia tree) is an antisenescent.

Only one potency is employed with gemmotherapeutic remedies in liquid form, that is 2X. Further research needs to be carried out to determine their efficacy at higher potencies and, with only twenty-nine remedies tested, more are needed to fully explore their potential. Dosages are rather high, bearing in mind that a 2X potency represents a relatively large material dose. Ten or fifteen drops on the tongue totalling fifty to seventy-five drops per day for periods up to two months are recommended.

Examples of successful gemmotherapeutic treatments on the results of clinical experience only (not provings) are as follows:

NERVOUS SYSTEM
Nerve tonic: **Betula verrucosa (seed) 2X**
Psychosomatic disorders: **Ficus carica (buds) 2X**
Sedative: **Tilia tomentosa (buds) 2X**
RESPIRATORY SYSTEM
Asthma: **Viburnum lantana (buds) 2X, Ribes nigrum (buds) 2X**
Emphysema: **Corylus avellana (buds) 2x, Ribes nigrum (buds) 2X**
Rhinopharynritis: Carpinus betula (buds) 2X
CARDIOVASCULAR AND CIRCULATORY SYSTEM

Venous circulation disorders: **Sorbus domesticus (buds) 2X, Castanea vesca (buds) 2X**

Cardiac disorders: **Crataegus oxycantha (buds) 2X**

DIGESTIVE SYSTEM

Stomach disorders: **Ficus caricus (buds) 2X**

Colitis: **Vaccinum vitis Idea (young shoots) 2X**

Constipation: **Vaccinum vitis Idea (young shoots) 2X, Betula pub. (buds) 2X, Quercus ped. (buds) 2X**

SKIN

Dry eczema: **Cedrus libani (young shoots) 2X**

WEEPING ECZEMA: **Ulmus campestre (buds) 2X**

ALLERGENS

Allergens are homoeopathic potencies of the causative substances of common allergies. Theoretically, any substance – animal, plant, mineral, foodstuffs or chemicals – known to cause an allergic reaction, whether inhaled, digested or in contact with the skin, eyes or mucous membranes, can be potentized by the normal Hahnemannian procedure and used prophylactically. In this context they may be seen as analogous to nosodes or isodes.

Commonly used allergens include Mixed Grass Pollen (pollen from twelve common species of grass), House Dust, House Dust Mite, Dog Hair, Cat Hair, Feathers, Wheat and Peanuts. Over two hundred allergens are now available.

In recent years, allergies considered to be the result of inhaling house dust are now ascribed to the house dust mite. This insect, invisible to the naked eye, infests carpets and linen. Even a new carpet may contain over one million mites per square metre, and a newly washed pillow, two or three thousand mites. It is believed that the microscopic faeces of the mite cause the allergic reaction.

The most popular allergen is Mixed Grass Pollen. It was subjected to a remarkably successful, randomized, double-blind, placebo-controlled clinical trial by Reilly, Taylor et al. in Scotland in 1986. The effects of Mixed Grass Pollen 30C given in tablet form were compared with placebo in 144 patients with active hay fever. The conventional design of the clinical trial followed a pilot study and earlier work of homoeopathic desensitization using potencies of House Dust Mite by Gibson, et al.

Participants had suffered from seasonal rhinitis for at least two years and were given Mixed Grass Pollen 30C or placebo on a double-blind basis for two weeks to check on homoeopathic aggravations and produce a base line for study. Pollen counts were taken in the vicinity of the trial on a daily basis and symptom scores were adjusted on the basis of a computerized statistical analysis.

The results proved conclusively that only the homoeopathically treated group of patients showed a clear reduction in their hay fever symptoms. As expected, initial aggravations were greater with those patients treated homoeopathically.

The report was published in *The Lancet* under the title, 'Is Homoeopathy a Placebo Response? Controlled Trial of Homoeopathic Potency with Pollen in Hayfever as Model'. It concluded, 'The drug used was potentized to the point where, in theory, none of the original material remained [see Avogadro's Hypothesis, Chapter 4]. These results offer no support for the suggestion that the observed effects were wholly due to the placebo response.'

An example of the importance of aetiology in homoeopathic practice and the efficacy of allergens concerned a male patient whose presenting symptoms were sinus problems with blockage in both nostrils, a feeling of suffocation, dry tongue, copious jelly-like, yellowish nasal discharge and a tickling, irritating cough. Aged sixty-two years, he had worked for sixteen years as a public swimming pool attendant and had retired four years before. Allopathic treatment with nasal decongestants since his retirement had brought only temporary relief. Diagnosis was allergic rhinitis.

On questioning, he admitted that the swimming pool where he worked was often heavily chlorinated but he got used to the smell, although he did suffer some eye and nose irritation at times in his early days.

I prescribed Chlorinum 30C tablets, three doses daily. After twenty-four days, at his follow-up consultation, he 'felt fine' and his symptoms were virtually cleared. His subsequent treatment was Chlorinum 30C at a reduced frequency of dosage of once daily on rising and he has had no problems since.

HOMOEOPATHIC DRAINAGE THERAPY

Drainage is an essential function of the body by which it frees or cleanses itself of the by-products of digestion, toxins, pollutants and the debris from the various processes of the body's metabolism. An example might be the waste from the repair of destroyed body tissue.

Drainage therapy or detoxification is defined as the therapeutic method of stimulating or regulating one or more of the natural excretory organs of the body. Drainage therapy activates or opens up the body's elimination channels and organs to enable optimum excretion of toxins from the body. The excretory organs are the liver, kidneys, lungs, skin, severed by the lymph vessels and mucous membranes.

Early forms of drainage were used in ancient times. The Greeks and Persians used massage systems to stimulate the lymph system. Turkish baths, sauna baths, herbal infusions, fasting, dieting, laxatives and modern diuretics and colonic irrigation, including enemas, the use of emetics and fasting, have all been used over the centuries.

It was Paracelsus the Swiss medical reformer who (in 1526) wrote, 'The quintessence is that which is abstracted from a substance and after it has been cleansed of all impurities it attains extraordinary powers and because of its purity it has the virtue to cleanse the body'. Studies by the French school included those of Leon Vannier who taught the doctrine of organic cleansing. He claimed that it was indispensable to homoeopathic treatment. Studies by Dr Nebel and Dr Tetau *et al.* confirmed Vannier's teachings. Dr Roy Matina of The Netherlands has stated 'in a clean body there can be no disease'. Health is the result of the natural ability of the body to detoxify itself physically, mentally and emotionally. Dr Maury, in his book *Drainage in Homoeopathy*, states that drainage is indispensable to obtain a clearly indicated remedy by the Law of Similars. Dr Maury sees drainage as a precursor to homoeopathic treatment whereby a patient is rendered more responsive to the correct remedy that is more accurately chosen by the application of the Law of Similars. Dr Bouko-Levy (1992) stated that the key to all treatment of chronic diseases is detoxification and it is the first condition necessary for a quick, complete healing.

In our modern society, with enviromental pollution and mental and emotional stresses, drainage therapy has never been more valid. Invasive polluting agents include atmospheric pollutants such as car exhaust fumes, lead, benzene and paraffin gases, nitrogen dioxide and sulphur dioxide, tobacco, alcohol, drugs, stimulants and even some constituents of dental fillings.

Ingested pollutants may include contaminated or decayed food and water, toxic additives in food products, poor diet, tobacco and some modern prescribed drugs.

Inhaled pollutants include smog, dust, tobacco smoke, nitrogen dioxide, sulphur dioxide, carbon dioxide, carbon monoxide, ozone, nitrogen and constituents of aerosol sprays.

Induced toxins are the result of mental and emotional influences, which interfere with the natural energy processes acting on the tissues, and include anxiety, worry, stress and shock. Induced toxins may also be the result of poor body hygiene.

The Functions of Drainage

The functions of drainage therapy are as follows:

1. The elimination of accumulated body toxins by the excretory organs.
2. Organic stimulation.
3. Reabsorption of a localized congestion.
4. Overall, drainage helps to maintain the normal balance between assimilation and catabolism.

Drainage may be direct, whereby the specific excretory organ such as the liver or the kidneys is directly stimulated, or indirect, whereby the endocrine system is stimulated to release hormones and other messages for opening up the drainage channels. Body toxins are eliminated through channels that offer the most convenient route of excretion

available. These channels are sweat, faeces, urine, menstrual flow, skin eruptions, tears, ear discharges, catarrhal discharges, nasal discharges and exhaled air, including carbon dioxide and nitrogen.

Simoneon suggested three steps are essential for detoxification:

1. dislodging or excreting toxins from the cell structure;
2. cleansing released toxins from the filtering organs; and
3. draining and eliminating toxins by the excretory organs and their removal from the body.

These processes are continous and the natural drainage function of the body is a continous process.

Toxification Symptoms

A clean system of connected tissues is a key factor to health. The intercellular system of connected tissue in the body can become clogged and rigid with stagnant toxins and metabolic waste products. A simple analogy is that of a car engine that requires servicing including a overdue oil change.

The general symptoms of toxification include drowsiness and lethargy, dullness, sluggishness, mental and physical fatigue, lack of concentration, loss of memory, skin complaints including rashes, boils, pimples and eczema, nausea, constipation, diarrhoea, pain in the area of the liver, moodiness, thickly coated tongue (white or yellow), bitter taste in the mouth, headaches, migraines, restlessness, dizziness, gout, insomnia, halitosis, poor appetite, flatulence, abdominal swelling, digestive problems, and dysfunction of the liver and gall-bladder, emphysema, premenstrual tension and profuse sweating.

Homoeopathic Drainage

The removal of the symptoms associated with the dysfunction of an excretory organ or organs and the removal of blockage of drainage channels is the prime objective of homoeopathic drainage. However, the many common symptoms associated with toxificaton of the body may confuse the practitioner in the choice of correct homoeopathic remedy according to the Similimum. Thus, clarification of a patient's symptom picture by drainage therapy that may be confusing to the practitioner, could be a precursor to homoeopathic treatment. The symptom picture then may enable the accurate prescription of the correct remedy for the underlying chronic condition.

Another advantage of drainage therapy prior to homoeopathic treatment is that it may reduce the likelihood of an aggravation during the homoeopathic treatment itself. Apart from the removal of the specific symptoms of detoxification, homoeopathic drainage can inculcate a feeling of general mental and physical well-being in a patient, which in turn will optimize the body's immune system.

A homoeopathic drainage programme will be enhanced if the treatment includes a proper diet with an adequate intake of vitamins and essential minerals and trace elements, relaxation, adequate exercise, breathing exercises and increase of water by drinking and perhaps sauna baths, a lymph massage and colonic irrigation.

A homoeopathic drainage programme using a classical, single, homoeopathic remedy is the simpliest approach. Homoeopathic drainage employs remedies that have an affinity-specific excretory organ or the channels that serve them. So, for example, for *liver* dysfunctions Chelidonium, Conium, Taraxacum, Solidago and Carduus mar. would be prescribed.

For the *kidneys* Formica rufa, Sarsaparilla, Solidago and Cholestrinum would be prescribed. For the *skin* the prescription would be Calendula, Petroleum, Fumaria and Viola tricolor. For the *lungs*, Sticta would be the remedy; for the *stomach*, Condurango or Ornithogallum. For the *pancreas*, Stella; for the *rectum*, Ruta grav., Scrofula and Senna. For the *uterus*, Thlaspi bursa and Helonias; for the *prostrate*, Chimaphilia; for the bladder, Physalis. The *mucous membranes* are treated with Hydrastis, Euphrasia, Sabadilla and Allium cepa.

Mode of action of Drainage Remedies

CARDUUS MAR.: Swelling of the liver, with the sensation of pressure on the liver, biliary calculi with extension to the right shoulder blade, right upper quadrant pain.

SOLIDAGO VIRGA: Has been described as 'a great old kidney medicine'. Very sensitive to kidney pressure, coated tongue (linked with urinary condition), bitter taste (especially at night), pain in abdomen on both sides of naval (especially) on deep pressure, diarrhoea, scanty and difficult urine, urine a dark brown colour (or reddish brown) with sediment, clear but 'stinking' urine (Bright's disease), urine contains blood, phosphate, slime and gravel of dead skin cells and mucous particles, kidney congestion, backache, blotches on hands and feet, itching and dropsy.

BERBERIS VULGARIS: A poor memory, incapable of sustained mental effort. Renal conditions, bubbling sensations in region of kidneys. Bladder affections. Dryness of eyes, nose and mouth. Vertigo on stooping. Headaches (sensation as if head encased in helmet), sensation of sand in eyelids, white tongue, sudden intense pain in liver region, nausea before breakfast, bitter taste in mouth, cramping pains around naval, burning, boiling pain on the left side, urine turbid with chalky white deposit or reddish, containing blood. Burning in urethra. Weariness, weakness, especially in lower limbs. Lumbago-type pains shooting down to low limbs. Sleep unrefreshing and tiredness during the day.

SCROPHULARIA NODOSA: Excessive drowsiness, constriction of chest. Painful, swollen piles, discharges from rectum, lower abdominal pain. Pain in liver, prickly itching all over the body. Vertigo. Drowsiness in morning, afternoon and after eating, eczema. Rancid taste in throat. Pain on pressure in liver region. Burning in urethra, frequent, scanty emission of urine. Prickly itching, worse on backs of hands.

LYCOPODIUM CLAVATUM: Flatulence, bitter taste in the mouth. Constipation. Increase in appetite, but easily satiated.

NUX VOMICA: Hypochondria, hepatic constriction and congestion, jaundice, nausea, gastro-intestinal dyspepsia, constipation, haemorrhoids. Abuse of all stimulants, for example alcohol and tobacco.

SENNA: Exhaustion through excess nitrogance waste. Laxative. Infantile colic (full of wind). Heaviness in head, particularly in stooping. Sweating, especially hands, exhaustion, coated tongue, constipation with muscular weakness, whole alimentary system sluggish, painful colic with suspended flatulence (especially children). Grumbling in abdomen, excessive deposits of urates in urine with increased specific gravity, enlarged and tender liver, prolapsed rectum with sore anus.

CHOLESTERINUM: Chronic enlargement of the liver, jaundice. Formation of gallstones.

SECALE CORNUTUM (ERGOT): Urine retention. Pale, drawn face. Sallow skin, dry and shrivelled or yellow and leathery. Confused thoughts. Urinary complaints and nausea. Weakness of intellectual capacity, nose bleeds, vertigo, hair loss, halitosis, yellowish tongue and tingling at the tip of tongue. Unnatural nervous appetite, nausea worse on eating, liver disorders, 'inflammation and gangrene' or enlarged liver, colic, offensive or watery diarrhoea. Scanty, hot, burning urine, numbness and twitching of the facial muscles, tingling of fingers and feet. Limbs feel heavy or even paralytic, staggering walk, shrivelled yellow skin with small boils and ulcers.

TARAXACUM: Diuretic, gastric headaches, red, sensitive tongue with a bitter taste. Profuse sweating at night, urination difficult.

COLOCYNTHIS: Cramp-like abdominal pain (relieved by strong pressure on abdomen and by bending double), gall-bladder, colic and cystitis.

Prescription

Homoeopathic drainage therapy may usually be completed in five to seven days. Drainage remedies are normally prescribed in low potencies such as 2X, 3X, 6X or 12X, or even as mother tincture (for example Berberis for kidney stones). The frequency of dosage is relatively high at three to four doses daily until the symptoms subside.

QUESTIONS

Answers are given on page

1. Hahnemann approved of prescribing more than one remedy in each case, providing:.

----

2. Arsenicum album and Nux vomica would not be used in a combination remedy because:--

3. The bowel nosodes were introduced by:

----

4. The classical homoeopathic remedy, which is most representative of each bowel nosode, is known as the:

----

5. The keynote for the following bowel nosodes is:

(a) Morgan Gaertner --
(b) Gaertner Bach --
(c) Sycotic Co. --

6. The basic principle of organotherapy is:

----

7. Low potencies--the activity of an organ or gland.

8. The 'blocking' of metallic ions in the body is caused by the chemical process of

----

9. The only potency employed to date in gemmotherapy is

----

10. State six symptoms of body toxification:

CHAPTER 10
Computers in Homoeopathy

*Homoeopathic practice administration.
Databases. Information exchange. Online
learning. Computerized repertorization.
Research.*

INTRODUCTION

Modern computer technology has provided
a sophisticated tool for homoeopathic
practice and research, and the personal
computer has, in the last decade of the
twentieth century, become an intrinsic part
of the whole infrastructure of homoeopathy.

The principal applications are set out
below.

HOMOEOPATHIC PRACTICE ADMINISTRATION

Patient records, clinical data, appointments
for consultations, financial records and
accounts, administrative data, correspondence, computer files etc.

DATABASES

1. Database systems for homoeopathic
   literature with precise details of the source

and reliability. One advanced system
developed in Europe is code named
RADAR (Rapid Aid To Drug Aimed
Research) and is used for clinical research.
Another advance has been *Reference
Works* which is provided as a support
to computerized repertorization. It
combines all the major *Materia Medicas*
and Repertories in one large source work,
including the Repertories of Kent,
Boericke, Clarke, Boenninghausen, Knerr,
Roberts, Ward and Murphy. Also included
are works such as Phatak's *Concise
Materia Medica*, Morrison's *Desktop
Guide* and Richardson-Boedler's *Bach
Remedies*. One click of the mouse can
raise all the information available on a
given topic.

2. Clinical databases involve the collection of
   data from thousands of actual cases in
   clinical practice. The Faculty of
   Homoeopathy in the UK has played a
   leading role in collecting this data, which
   ranges from recording remedies to treat
   simple complaints to sophisticated data on
   homoeopathic consultations with full case
   histories, the analysis of which may be
   used to test our asssumptions on the
   selection of homoeopathic remedies.
   Had computers been available during
   nearly two hundred years of successful
   homoeopathic clinical cases, there can be

no doubt that we would by now have had overwhelming proof of its efficacy.

EXCHANGE OF INFORMATION

With the development of the Internet and e-mail world-wide, there is a constant flow of information on homoeopathic theory and practice, and it provides a striking vehicle for debate.

Homeonet is one such computer network and is a forum for homoeopaths to share information and news on a world-wide basis.

ONLINE LEARNING

The entire learning process may now be facilitated by computers. Online students of homoeopathy using CD-Rom can receive one-to-one guidance electronically twenty-four hours a day, seven days a week.

Another example is the Online Study Group established by the British Institute of Homoeopathy in 1998. The first of its kind, it provides a facility for all graduates and students of the Institute in seventy-two different countries to participate in animated discussions on a wide range of homo-eopathic topics and exchange information. Students can communicate with their personal tutors by e-mail, using PC or Mac machines. The British Institute website is www.britinsthom.com.

COMPUTERIZED REPERTORIZATION AND SERVICES

For speed and accuracy nothing can match the use of computers as a tool for repertorizing. Great progress has been made in this field and there are now several excellent programs available, which can scan entire repertories or a combination of several Repertories in seconds to give a graded choice of matching remedies on the classical pattern. The main programs are the MacRepertory, the RADAR system, the CARA program and the HOMPATH. Each system provides an accurate computer repertory function plus special features for analysis and research.

CARA Program

This excellent programme permits the homoeopathic practitioner to select the full Kent Repertory, the Boericke Repertory or other Repertories. By simple keystrokes, one can move through the Repertories at will, returning to the beginning through the exit key.

The computer analyses the symptoms and scans the Repertories awarding 'scores': three stars for a **black type** remedy of the highest grade, two stars for a remedy printed in *italics* and one star for plain type entries. The programme is designed to gather and analyse symptoms, and provides additional facilities for remedy analysis.

Several improved versions of the CARA programme have been introduced over the years, each with many new features. CARA Pro for Windows 95 presents a new computerized Repertory and *Materia Medica*. New combined Repertories are provided, which include those in the Synthetic Repertory.

Other features include several *Materia Medicas* and an acute prescriber. Cases can be analysed directly against the *Materia Medica*, providing a unique feature for the accurate selection of the Simillimum remedy.

MacRepertory Program

The very popular MacRepertory is arguably

the easiest-to-use and most powerful repertory program. MacRepertory was created by classical homeopaths and graphic designers instead of computer programmers so it works in the way that homeopaths intuitively do. It enables you to quickly find and analyse your patient's symptoms using over nineteen Repertories and then to verify your thoughts quickly in two dozen *Materia Medicas.*

The repertory on the screen looks just like the book that you are used to. The remedies are in plain, italic or bold and the indenting is preserved. The familiar format makes it easy to switch from the book to the computer.

The repertorial library is very broad, with Allen, Boericke, Boenninghausen, Clarke, Knerr, Roberts, Ward, Richardson-Boedler's Bach, Eizayaga's Disease Algorithms, Murphy's Medical Repertory, the Complete Repertory, the Phoenix, Scholten's Themes, etc.

To collect rubrics for an analysis you just point the mouse at the rubric and click. Another click and the rubrics are analysed.

The program comes configured with a variety of tried-and-trusted models for analysing cases. Each model emphasizes different aspects of the case: certain sections of the repertory, rubrics that contain particular words, rubrics with nosodes, the rare remedies that do surprisingly well, the remedies that have keynotes in the case, or the remedies that simply cover the most symptoms.

You can also find remedies based on their relationships to the most prominent families in the case: that is Cenchris when snakes are doing well. Or you can find the salts made from the highest scoring remedies: that is Calcarea sulphuricum and Hepar sulph. when Calcarea and Sulphur run through the case.

MacRepertory displays the results of your analysis in a variety of colour graphs that make the most likely remedies clear. The graphs run the gamut from straightforward, with a bar graph showing how well each remedy fits the case, to visionary, with a rainbow graph that displays each family and where it fits into the evolution of life. The coloured bars of the bar graph show how highly each remedy scores and indicate in which kingdom it belongs. The waffle graph simultaneously displays rubrics and remedies in a clear, concise format. The city graph offers a vibrant, bird's-eye view of the rubrics and leading remedies. The scientifically inclined will appreciate the scatter graph; strategies are plotted in four dimensions by combining two axes with dot size and colour.

MacRepertory has included graphs to help you look at families of remedies. Up until now we have had to consider each remedy one at a time. In science when you want to identify something unknown you look for its similarity to a known group and then choose between members of that group. For the first time in the history of homeopathy you can examine a case and find the families of remedies that best cover the symptoms. Then remedy selection becomes a matter of selecting the closest fitting member of the family.

The remedies are organized into more than seven hundred botanical, chemical and biological families. Beside the traditional kingdoms there are other ways of organizing remedies: miasms; five elements; plant chemicals; Vega's boxes; Murphy's planets; Boyd's types, etc. To illustrate the possibilities, imagine analysing a case and discovering that the Solanaceae family covers the symptoms very well. You remember that this family is known for its ability to cause nervous symptoms, which is indeed the centre of your case. Now, with a single click,

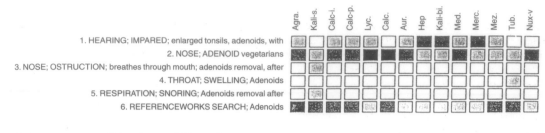

Macrepertory Display of Results

display just those remedies in the Solanaceae plant family; then simply choose between Bell., Caps., Dulc., Hyos., Stram., Tab., etc.

There is a special set of graphs especially to illuminate the families. For example, the plant, animal and periodic tables show exactly which plants, animals or elements are prominent in your case. When you click on a family's square you'll see the case's rubrics limited to only the remedies in that family.

Click on the 'Na' square to see every Natrum found in the case. Or in the plant chart click on the carrot to see all the remedies made from roots. Or in the animal chart select the picture of the snake to limit the graph to the snakes. If you need even more choices you can create your own graphs. You can combine graph styles with statistics, fonts, transparencies, planes, labels, rubrics, strategies and clipboards to create just the graph you want and save it as a convenient button on the screen. Once you're close to a decision, MacRepertory can make the choice clearer by limiting the graphs to groups of remedies. You can limit the remedies shown in the graphs to members of a particular family (such as snakes, plants, milks, gases, nuts or Ranunculaceae, etc.). Hide all the polycrests if you would like to highlight lesser known remedies or display only those remedies found in selected rubrics, etc.

You can also find any word or combination of words in the Repertory. You could find every rubric concerning pregnancy, chagrin, joy, haemoptysis or catalepsy. Then you could repertorize the results. You can also search for remedies in the entire Repertory or a single section. You can choose to see only the most unique symptoms of a remedy. And using the search you can discover symptoms common to families of remedies, i.e. the spiders. You can save information about the patient, analysis, diagnoses, plan, prescription, billing, lab reports, remedy's effect, aggravation, etc. This information can be used in database programs for mailing lists, billings or research on homoeopathy, etc. You can easily make additions to the Repertories and *Materia Medica* that come in the program.

MacRepertory is sold in three configurations so, no matter what your commitment to homoeopathy, there is a program that will help you to prescribe more effectively.

Reference Works

Reference Works is a ground-breaking program that combines the completeness of the *Materia Medicas* with the ease of finding rubrics in the Repertory and the analysis power of a repertorial program. First of all Reference Works is a huge library with more than 390 volumes of *Materia Medica*: all the way from the *Materia Medicas* of Allen, Boericke, Clarke and

Kent to Morrison, Vermeulen and Scholten. There are hundreds of provings, including the work of Sherr, Herrick, Promethius, Eising and Müller, together with tens of thousands of articles from such journals as the *British Homeopathic Journal*, *The Homoeopath* and links and cured cases from homeopaths such as Mangialavori, Italiano, Gray, Heron, etc.

With Repertories you often cannot find the most unique aspects of the patient in repertory language, but with Reference Works you can search for the patient's exact words. This can lead to more precise prescribing. Reference Works enables you to instantly find a patient's symptoms anywhere that they may be hidden in the *Materia Medicas* and Repertories. For example, a search through the entire library for 'jealousy' took a single second and found 1,298 references to 227 remedies – compare that with Murphy's Repertory, for example, where there are only 35 remedies known.

Once you have found that special symptom you can browse through the descriptions of remedies from a wide range of books much more easily than ever before. The program displays every reference to the symptom in a list; a click on any reference instantly opens the *Materia Medica* to the full text with your symptom underlined. Pressing the tab key leaps you to the next reference. Unlike real books you can jump directly from the mind symptoms of Apis in one book to the mind symptoms of Apis in another or from the mind section in Stramonium to the mind section in Hyoscymus.

You can collect interesting information from several *Materia Medicas* to print out for your personal *Materia Medica*, a lecture or the patient's chart. Once you have found every reference in the *Materia Medica* to the patient's symptoms, Reference Works can analyse the results as though they were from a Repertory. Reference Works adds up the occurrences of the symptom in each remedy and draws a graph of the highest scoring remedies. Where there are grades in the *Materia Medica* (as there are in Hering, Allen, etc.) they are taken into account in the analysis. You can export the results of any search to MacRepertory where they can be used as rubrics in a repertorial case analysis. Reference Works is sold in three configurations based on the size of the libraries.

NOTE: *The Gift of Homeopathy* CD available, inter alia, from the British Institute of Homoeopathy, includes simple versions of MacRepertory and ReferenceWorks, along with two additional programs. It was generously donated to the homoeopathic community as a fundraiser for non-profit organizations and thousands of pounds have found their way to worthy organizations through this gift.

RADAR Program

The RADAR program (currently RADAR 6.0 for Windows) is an IBM program claimed to be a new generation of software. It provides the Synthesis, an expanded Repertory facility including the Kent Repertory in an identical format, plus many additions from other Repertories. There is sufficient spread for the display of some rubrics with only a few remedies to have the remedies on the same line, but for most rubrics a number indicates how many remedies are contained within them. However, a single keystroke displays all the remedies.

A particular page from the Repertory may be displayed if required, or even a column. Typing the selected rubric or sub-rubric will display all those listed. Up to six key works

197

may be included in any search for the most accurately selected rubric and the program quickly scans the entire Repertory.

Symptoms can be graded in the range 0 to 10. A zero grade will exclude that rubric from the repertorization and by changing the selected symptoms a single list of rubrics may be analysed in several different ways.

VES (Vithoulkas Expert System, Version 2) is a special feature of the RADAR program. It enables the practitioner to view the analytical function and knowledge in a specialized area to evaluate the symptoms in depth. Consistent with Dr George Vithoulkas's approach, mental and emotional symptoms are given prominence. Cases may be analysed with no limit to the number of symptoms and a 'homoeopathic' or alphabetical order in the Repertory may be selected.

Like the MacRepertory and CARA programs, the RADAR program is undergoing constant updating and improve-ments, which suggest that we have not yet reached the optimum level of an already sophisticated computer facility. The scope is truly limitless.

Research

Computerized studies of complex molecular and electronic configurations from the nucleii to infinity may shed more light on the nature of liquid high potencies above the Avogadro Limit, where theoretically none of the original molecules of the mother tincture exist.

Supercomputers are capable of providing a more sophisticated interpretation of the evidence produced by research with nuclear magnetic resonance spectographic analysis (NMR) – see Chapter 4.

It is clear that the future progress of homoeopathy during the twenty-first century is inexorably tied to computer technology.

Bibliography

Cook, Trevor *Samuel Hahnemann: His Life & Times*
(Thorsons, 1981). (Third Edition 2000, British Institute
of Homoeopathy).

Dudgeon, R.E. *Life & Work of Samuel Hahnemann*
1854

Haehl, *Richard Samuel Hahnemann, His Life & Work*
(Leipzig, 1922)

Hahnemann, Samuel *The Chronic Diseases, Their
Peculiar Nature & Their Homeopathic Cure*
(Boerick & Tafel, Philadelphia, 1896)

Cook, Trevor *Homeopathic Medicine Today: A
Modern Course of Study*
(Keats, USA, 1987)

Hahnemann, Samuel *Organon of Medicine*
(Kunzli, Gollancz, UK, 1989)

Hahnemann, Samuel *Organon of the Medical Art*
(Translation by Steven Decker, Birdcage, USA, 1996)

Zandvoort, Roger *The Complete Repertory*
(Inst. for Research in Homeopathic Info. &
Symptomatology, Holland, 1996)

Clarke, J.H. *Dictionary of the
Materia Medica* (3 Volumes)
(Jain, India)

Verspoor, R., *Homoeopathy Renewed: Cure & Prevention
of Chronic Disease*
(Norsana Academy, 1998)

Kent, J.T. *Repertory of Materia Medica*
(Jain, India)

Kent, J.T. *Lectures on Homeopathic Philosophy*
(Jain, India)

Allen, H.C. *Keynotes with Nosodes*

Allen, K. *Repertory Workbook & Solution Guide*

Roberts, H. *Principles & Art of Cure*
(Jain, India)

Gibson, D. *Studies of Homeopathic Remedies*
(Beaconsfield, 1987, UK)

Verma & Vaid *Encyclopedia of Homeopathic
Pharmacopoeia* (Volumes 1&2)
(Jain, India, 1997)

Weekes & Bullen *Bach Flower Remedies*
(C. W. Daniel, UK)

Boericke & Dewey *The Twelve Tissue Salts of Schuessler*
(Jain, India)

Ullman, Dana *Homeopathic Medicine for Children &
Infants* (Penguin Putnam, USA)

Blackie, Margery *Classical Homoeopathy*
(Beaconsfield, UK, 1990)

Paterson, John *The Bowel Nosodes* (Brit.Hom.J., UK,
1936)

Maury, E.A. *Drainage In Homoeopathy*
(Daniel, UK, 1982)

Clarke, J.H. *A Clinical Repertory to the Dictionary of
Materia Medica*
(Jain, India)

Shepherd, D. *Magic of the Minimum Dose*
(Daniel, UK)

Morrison, R. *Desktop Companion to Physical Pathology*
(Hahnemann Clinic Publishing, USA, 1998)

Roberts, H. *Sensations. As If*
(Jain, India)

Macleod, George *A Veterinary Materia Medica*
(Daniel, UK)

Logan, Robin *Homeopathic Treatment of Eczema*
(Beaconsfield, UK, 1998)

Chakravarty, Anima *Homeopathic Drug Personalities*
(Jain, India)

Coulter, Catherine *Portraits of Homeopathic Medicines*
(Volumes 1&2) USA, 1993, (Quality Medical
Publishing)

Moskowitz, Richard *Homeopathic Medicines for
Pregnancy & Childbirth* (North Atlantic Books, 1992)

Verspoor, R. *A Time For Healing: Origins & Treatment
of Chronic Illness* (1995)

Close, Stuart *The Genius of Homeopathy*
(B. Jain, India, 1993)

Julian, O *Materia Medica of New Homoeopathic
Remedies*
(Beaconsfield, UK)

Useful Addresses

HOMOEOPATHIC BOOKS

Homoeopathic Educational Services
2124 Kittredge Street
Berkeley
CA 94704
USA

Minerva Books
173 Fulham Palace Road
London W6 8QT
England

The Minimum Price Books
250 High Street
PO Box 2187
Blaine
WA 98231
USA

British Institute of Homoeopathy
Cygnet House
Market Square
Staines
Middlesex TW18 4RH
England

Ainsworths Homoeopathic
Pharmacy
36 Cavendish Street
London W1M 7LH
England

Homoeopathic Books
520 Washington Blvd
Suite 423
Marina Del Rey
CA 90292
USA

Awesome Book Company
52 Dollis Park
Finchley
London N3 1BS, England

HOMOEOPATHIC ORGANIZATIONS

Homeopathic Medical Association
6 Livingstone Road
Gravesend
Kent DA12 5DZ
England

Society of Homoeopaths
2 Artizan Road
Northampton
NN1 4HU
England

Faculty of Homoeopathy
Great Ormond Street
London WC1N 3HR
England

American Institute of Homoeopathy
925E 17th Avenue
Denver
CO 80218
USA

National Association of
Homoeopathic Groups
11 Wingle Tye Road
Burgess Hill
RH15 9HR
England

National Center for Homoeopathy
(USA)
801 North Fairfax Street
Suite 306
Alexandria
VA 22314
USA

National United Professional
Association of Trained
Homoeopaths

1445 St Joseph Blvd
Gloucester
ON KIC 7K9
Canada

HOMOEOPATHIC REMEDIES

Ainsworths Homoeopathic
Pharmacy
36 Cavendish Street
London W1M 7LH
England

Weleda (UK) Limited
Heanor Road
Ilkeston
Derbyshire
England

Helios Homoeopathic Pharmacy
89–97 Camden Road
Tunbridge Wells
Kent TN1 2QR
England

Dolisos America Inc
3014 Rigel Avenue
Las Vegas
NV 89102
USA

Galen Homoeopathics
Lewell Mill
West Stafford
Dorchester
Dorset DT2 8AN
England

Luyties Pharmacal Company
4200 Laclede Ave
PO Box 8080
St Louis
MO 63156–8080
USA

Boericke Tafel Inc
1011 Arch Street
Philadelphia 19107
USA

Dolisos Inc
1240 Rue Beaumont
No. 6 Mount Royal
Quebec H3P 3E5
Canada

Santa Monica Homoeopathic
Pharmacy
629 Broadway
Corner of 7th Street
Santa Monica
CA 90401
USA

**HOMOEOPATHIC
JOURNALS**

Student Homoeopath
191a Kentish Town Road
Kentish Town
London NW5 2JU
England

Homoeopathy International
Published by: HMA (UK)
6 Livingstone Road
Gravesend
Kent DA12 5DZ
England

British Homeopathic Journal
Published by: Faculty of
Homoeopathy
Hahnemann House

2 Powis Place
Great Ormond Street
London WC1N 3HT
England

International Newsletter
Published by: British Institute of
Homoeopathy
Cygnet House
Market Square
Staines
Middlesex TW18 4RH
England

Homeopathy Today
Published by: NCH
801 North Fairfax St, Suite 306
Alexandria
VA 22314
USA

Answers to Questions

CHAPTER 1

1. Cinchona officinalis.
2. 1779.
3. Purging.
4. Organon of the Healing Art/Organon of Rational Healing Organon of Medicine/The Organon.
5. Provings.
6. Lachesis, Hepar sulphuris, Theridion, Spigelia.
7. Swedenborg.
8. Typhoid fever.
9. Père Lachaise Cemetery.
10. Iatrogenic disease.

CHAPTER 2

1. Like suffering. Like disease. Similar suffering.
2. Artificial disease.
3. 'Other therapy'.
4. Arndt–Schultz.
5. Complex disease.
6. Dynamis.
7. Proving symptoms.
8. Vital force.
9. Dr Edward Jenner.
10. Subtle spirit. Life field. Morphogenic field. Biological closed circuitry

CHAPTER 3

1. Plant: Poison nut tree
   Animal: Blister beetle

(Spanish fly)
Plant: Poison ivy
Sea animal: Cuttlefish.
Squid
Snake: Bushmaster.
Surucu
Element: Metal
2. Calcium carbonate.
   Calcium sulphide.
   Potassium dichromate.
   Sodium chloride (salt).
   Silver nitrate.
3. Arsen alb., Belladonna, Aconite, Pulsatilla, Nux vomica,
   Rhus tox., Sulphur, Calc. carb., Graphites, Lycopodium,
   Sepia officinalis and others.
4. Decimal X.
   Centesimal C.
   Millesimal m (or mm).
   Fifty millesimal LM.
5. 1: 10
   1: 100
   1: 1,000
   1: 50,000
6. 4X 1×10^{-4}
   2C 1×10^{-4}
   30X 1×10^{-30}
   24C 1×10^{-48}
8. Hard tablets: Lactose (80%)/Sucrose (20%), machine compressed.
   Soft tablets: Lactose (100%), hand compressed.
9. X. L. M.

CHAPTER 7

1. 3, 6, 12, 24, 30, 60.
2. Units or sub-units of 12.
3. Cinchona officinalis.
4. Art.
5. Chromium, manganese, selenium, copper, cobalt, zinc, iodine, lithium, boron, molybdenum, vanadium.
6. Calcarea causticum (caustica).
7. Calcium hydroxide and Potassium sulphate.
8. Hexagons (six-sided).

CHAPTER 9

1. The remedies must not be given at the same time.
2. The remedies antidote one another.
3. Dr John Paterson, Dr Elizabeth Paterson, Dr Edward Bach.
4. Prototype remedy.
5. (*a*) Congestion.
   (*b*) Malnutrition.
   (*c*) Irritability.
6. The organ acts upon the organ.
7. Stimulate.
8. Chelation.
9. 2X.

Remedy Index

Index

A

Abbreviations in homoeopathy 51
Abrotanum 103, 119
Aconitum napellus 120
Aetiology 35, 187
Aggravation 66, 70
Allium cepa 40–1
Alumina 41, 121
AIDS 23
Allergens 86, 187
Allopathy 28
American Institute of Homoeopathy 12
Analysis of homoeopathic medicines 53
Apis mellifica 122
Anthrocinum 12
Antim. tart. 12
Antipsoric remedies 59, 61
Antisycotic remedies 61
Antisyphilitic remedies 61
Applied homoeopathy 175
Argentum nitricum 123
Aristotle 27
Arndt, Rudolf 32
Arnica montana 124
Arsenicum album 125
Artificial disease 30
Artemisia annua 103
Artemisia vulgaris 103
Arum triphyllum 61
Asafoetida 61
Aurum metallicum 42, 126
Avogadro's Hypothesis 48, 64

B

Bach, Dr Edward 176
Bacillus No. 7 178, 182
Belladonna 127
Berberis vulgaris 128, 190
Biochemic remedies 86

Bioenergies 33
Biological remedies 42
Biotherapies 182
Biphasic response curve 32
Blackie, Dr Margery 35, 62, 85
Bloodletting 8
Bonninghausen, Carl 15
Borax 109
Bowel nosodes 176
British Institute of Homoeopathy 194
Broussais, Dr 8
Bryonia alba 129
Bufo rana 41

C

Calcarea carbonica 130
Calcarea caustica 110
Calcarea fluorica 132
Calcarea phosphorica 106
Calcarea sulphurica 106
Calendula officinalis 43
Cantharis 134
Carcinosin 60
Carbo vegetabilis 135
CARA program 194
Care of homoeopathic remedies 55
Caulophyllum 40, 136
Cell salts 105
Centesimal series of potencies 44–5
Chain, Ernst 22
Chamomilla 137
Chelation 185
Chelidonium majus 190
Chimaphilia 190
Cholestrinum 191
Chromium oxydatum 109
Chronic Diseases, The 35, 68
Churchill, Winston 22
Cinchona officinalis 6–7, 27,

40
Clarus, Professor 18, 31
Classical homoeopathy 71
Cobaltum metallicum 108
Cocculus indicus 138
Colchicum autumnale 41
Complete Repertory 76
Complex disease 30
Computers in homoeopathy 193
Computerized repertorization 194
Concomitant treatment 87
Conium maculatum 139
Creams 52
Crocus sativus 121
Cuprum aceticum 108
Cuprum metallicum 140
Cupping 8

D

Databases 193
Decimal series of potencies 44
Decker, Steven 199
Dechelation 185
Declaration of Geneva 88
Depth of symptoms 75
Detoxification 189
Detweiler, Dr 12
Differential diagnosis 73
Dilutions 44–49
Disraeli, Benjamin 21
Doctrine of Signatures 109
Drainage therapy 86, 188
Dresden 9, 16
Drosera rotundifolia 41, 141
Drug affinities 116
Drug pictures 116
Dudley, Dr Pemberton 24
Dynamis 33
Dynamization 43
Dys. Co. 178, 182